STO

ALLEN COUNTY PUBLIC LIBRARY

ACPL ITEM
DISCAR

YO-BST-897

3.16.79

LIVING LONGER AND BETTER
Guide to Optimal Health

LIVING LONGER AND BETTER

Guide to Optimal Health

Harold Elrick, M.D.,
James Crakes, Ph.D., Sam Clarke, M.S.

0 048

79 9591 4

©1978 by
World Publications
Mountain View, CA 94042

No information may be reprinted in any
form without permission from the publisher.

Library of Congress 78-366
ISBN 0-89037-125-3

Acknowledgments

We wish to express our appreciation and gratitude to the following individuals for their valuable assistance in the preparation of this book: Ruth Walters, Ph.D., R.D.; Sharon Sveningson, R.D.; Linda Doninelli, R.D.; Harvey Selvestone, MSW; Donna Crakes; Willard Stevens, Ph.D.; and many friends, students, patients, family, who contributed suggestions, comments, and ideas for the book.

2050124

Contents

Introduction

The role of the physician has often been defined as twofold: He should prevent illness, and he should cure it when it occurs. Modern medicine has been preoccupied with the latter, while the former has been neglected.

As long as the physician is remunerated for curing illness rather than preventing it, his major efforts will be aimed in this direction. This is apparently what the public wants and what society supports. The physician almost never sees the healthy patient, and when such examinations do occur, they are almost always directed toward a search for the early signs of disease. Yet once disease exists, there is often little the physician can do to limit its progression. Rather than investigating for diseases that may be inadequately treatable, physicians must strive for a condition of health that will be totally incompatible to the formation of disease.

The authors of *Living Longer and Better: A Guide to Optimal Health* take a positive attitude on prevention. They regard optimal health as the antidote for illness, and optimal health is something that requires work to achieve. Their view of preventive health maintenance is not the casual annual checkup refrain "Lose twenty pounds and stop the smoking. Good day." They firmly believe that the physician and his health team must educate the patient to improve his style of living and to achieve the goal of optimal health.

This is not an approach we physicians are taught in medical schools. It is not the proselytizing of the faddist and the cultist. The authors have strong beliefs on the living habits necessary to achieve optimal health, and they provide the best available knowledge to support their position.

This area has so long been the province of the health cultist, it is encouraging that three such highly qualified professionals have made this effort to provide both the evidence for their views and a very practical health guide for the layman and the physician.

Alexander Leaf, M.D.

Dr. Leaf is Jackson Professor of Clinical Medicine, Harvard Medical School. He is also Chief of Medical Services, Massachusetts General Hospital.

Special Introduction

Many books have been written on health, starting in antiquity. One of the best was *Regiment of Helthe* written about a thousand years ago. This book so impressed King Henry VIII that it was translated into English and published in 1542. Much has also been written about preventive medicine, but mostly in a very dull fashion or unscientifically. Most books on diet and exercise are too detailed or so limited to the authors' special interests that they are not useful for many who, as individuals, vary greatly in age, strength, inherited aptitude, customs, and personal interests.

The contents of this book intrigue me; they have a pleasant variety of advice that can suit the individual case. Several special conditions besides the so-called "norm" are discussed, especially obesity, which in many cases is a real disease inadequately investigated until now.

Other important considerations discussed from the standpoint of nutrition and diet are diabetes, hypertension, atherosclerosis, uremia, and other edematous states. Helpful diets and recipes are included. The discussion of snacks interested me, for I have found that five or six properly arranged small snacks can be substituted for the usual three meals a day, similar to the finding that fowl are healthier when pecking their food than when stuffing themselves periodically.

This book is well-written, and should prove valuable to overfed and underexercised people all over the world.

Paul Dudley White, M.D.

Authors' Note: Dr. Paul Dudley White was America's most distinguished cardiologist. He lectured, wrote, and advised patients on prevention of heart disease for fifty years. He was a firm believer in regular exercise and proper eating habits. Furthermore, he practiced what he preached all his life. He remained very vigorous mentally and physically until his death on October 31, 1973 at the age of 87. A few months before his death, he reviewed the first draft of this book, and graciously wrote the above.

Part One:
Concepts for
the Coming Age

1
Optimal
Health

This book is about a different concept of health, and about living habits that can give you substantial protection against the major killers of our time: heart attacks, strokes, and other degenerative diseases. Your living habits affect the length of your life *and* the quality as well. Invigorating health is within your reach; it requires only your understanding and your commitment.

Prevention vs. Treatment

Before describing this new concept of health, let us examine prevailing medical education and practice. Current medical practice is oriented almost exclusively to the detection and treatment of disease. Almost all of our national health resources, physicians, research institutes, hospitals, and vast sums of money are directed towards the *cure* of disease. We pay our doctors to find and treat our sickness, *not to prevent it.* To the public, preventive medicine is annual check-ups and immunization against infectious diseases. To be sure, the over-weight patient receives advice to take off a few pounds, and the Surgeon General has declared "smoking is dangerous to your health," but preventive medicine is restricted for the most part to early detection of disease rather than reducing the causes of disease.

A medical philosophy oriented to treating detectable diseases was quite appropriate to the age of rampant infectious diseases; it is quite obsolete today when infections account for only 4% of the deaths and where "detectable disease" means a relatively advanced state of the disease. Application of therapy at such a point is simply too late.

There is a story that illustrates the failure of current medical practices to deal with modern medical problems. A well-trained young physician was walking along a river bank when he heard a cry for help from a drowning man in the river. Without hesitation the physician dived into the river, rescued the man, and resuscitated him with great skill. Just as he completed this deed there was another distress cry from another drowning person. The physician repeated the rescue operation with equal skill and efficiency. Then, a third drowning victim appeared.

At this moment another physician walked by and observed the situation. He said, "Why do you suppose so many people are falling into the river?" Whereupon the first physician shouted, "Don't bother me with your questions now. Don't you see I have no time to talk about such things?" and then dived into the water to rescue the next victim.

The first physician represents the conventional, well-trained practitioner who devotes his entire energies to the patchwork and emergency role that is required in most major adult diseases. This has proved neither effective nor rewarding in the long run, as evidenced by the mortality figures of our major diseases. The second physician is concerned with disease prevention, the only effective way to control the major diseases we are faced with today.

Cultivation of an exceptional level of health has received low priority by the physician, the medical educator, and thus by the public. But we are beginning to develop a new awareness that good health is more than "not being sick," that we cannot relinquish all responsibility for our own health to doctors. We see this in the spread of health food stores across the country, in the "jogging phenomenon," and in the proliferation of books on nutrition, weight control, and exercise directed to the general public.

Are these movements justified? Heart attacks and strokes were the causes of 900,000 deaths in the U.S. in 1975—more than 50% of all deaths. The risk factors for these diseases are similar: faulty diet, sedentary life, high blood pressure, smoking. Life expectancy has remained virtually the same for the past generation despite enormous sums of money solicited and spent in the hope and promise of extending lifespan.[1] Coronary care units, heart operations, and the various therapies for cancer have reached an incredible cost per patient, yet only to postpone death a few months or at most a few years. Results from these massive efforts are so small as to be undetectable in death rate statistics.

The key role of prevention is demonstrated in the fact that *60% of heart attack victims die before reaching a medical facility.*

Optimal vs. Normal Health Standards

The disease-treatment orientation is perpetuated in part by the interpretation generally given to "normal" test results. First, such tests are believed to distinguish between disease and health. Certainly, an abnormal finding does suggest illness; the error is made in believing that a normal finding implies health. For example, we now know that atherosclerosis (hardening of the arteries), the primary basis of heart disease, must be quite far advanced before it presents symptoms or evidence of disease. Most heart attacks result from a gradual build-up of fatty deposits (atherosclerotic plaques) in the arteries of the heart over many years before the heart attack. The disease may send no signals until the day the heart attack occurs. The patient unfortunately assumes from the "normal" test findings that he or she is free of this disease.

Relying on conventional testing or "feeling normal" as assurance of freedom from coronary heart disease is a mistake because *the accepted "normal" values or ranges are suspect.* These values are based on surveys of presumed healthy Americans, and this is a population with a high incidence of obesity, hypertension, and smoking; a poor level of physical fitness; and a diet that favors the development of atherosclerosis and diabetes.

We can illustrate the error of reliance on "normal" ranges with blood cholesterol. Cholesterol is generally regarded as one of the best measures for assessing risk of premature coronary heart disease. Studies on large numbers of apparently healthy Americans have shown a range of 150–300 mg%, and this is the range that is commonly used by laboratories and doctors as representing normal or healthy. Yet we know that the risk of cardiovascular disease increases progressively with any increase in blood cholesterol over 175 mg%. For example, at 300 mg% the risk is approximately four times as high as the risk at 175 mg%.[2]

We can see, then, that the public has little reason for assurance that its health is protected. On the contrary, depending on the normalcy concept has fostered false confidence.

We propose a different concept of health and medical practice more fitting to these times, to the public, and to the physician. We call this concept *Euexia* (Pronounced you-ex-eeya), an ancient Greek word used by Hippocrates and Aristotle meaning "good health" or "good habit of body." This word comes closest to expressing our concept of the highest or *optimal* state of health, fitness, and living habits. The aim of *Euexia* is not normalcy, but "optimalcy"; for only the optimal can provide assurance of the highest level of health. Only optimal standards can show the individual what he should aim for. Only a concept of optimal health can shake us out of our false assumptions and rigid habits.

What exactly do we mean by "optimal"? We mean using as our standards the highest reachable level in the physical, biochemical, and physiological tests in general use. These optimal standards have been derived from studies of selected populations, namely those with:

• The highest levels of cardiovascular-pulmonary fitness, such as competition distance runners.

• The lowest rates of cardiovascular and other degenerative diseases.

• The longest vigorous lifespan.

We find that these populations, which excel in physical work performance, freedom from disease, and longevity are similar in many physical and biochemical characteristics. The test results of these population groups have become the basis for our optimal standards.

The purpose of this book is to describe these optimal standards, optimal lifestyles, and health practices. We hope to help you attain your highest level of health, mental and physical vigor, and enjoyment of life.

Basic Tenets

"Optimal" is intended to mean the best achievable level for any given individual, i.e., his or her personal best. In some areas (blood pressure, heart rate, blood cholesterol) the optimal level is similar for everyone. In other areas (physical performance) it differs for each individual, because of genetic endowment or previous training.

• Optimal goals (standards) have been or can be established in all parameters of health-fitness and performance. These new standards should replace the normal standards as goals to aim for.

• *You*—not fate, the physician, heredity, the environment, or society—are primarily responsible for your level of health-fitness, which diseases you contract, how you respond to illness, and your lifespan.

• Your daily living habits determine your state of health-fitness.

• The living habits most important to health-fitness are those associated with eating, smoking, physical exertion, relaxing, and life situations (job, family, people, etc.).

• Regular use of a skill (ability, function, or muscle) results in the retention of that skill despite increasing age. Conversely, lack of use inevitably results in loss of the skill. *Disuse is the main cause of deterioration of physical and mental powers with increase in age.*

• The potential for improvement in all aspects of health-fitness with systematic use of proper conditioning methods is very great, regardless of age. In general, the younger the starting age the higher the level of health-fitness attainable.

• Quality of life (zest for life) is closely related to the level of health-fitness.

• The all-out effort of competition with self or peers, on a regular basis, in the healthy and conditioned individual, is a powerful motivating tool in achieving optimal goals, and speeds the process.

Derivation of Normal Standards

We live in a world of the "normal." We are expected to dress normally, pursue normal vocations, eat normally, and raise normal children. Everything we do is compared to a normal standard. Normal standards are derived from a statistical analysis of a population sample, which is used for describing a particular group and may not apply to individuals in other groups. Individuals used for this analysis are generally chosen because they are readily available for testing and because they are not obviously ill. Laboratory workers and insurance policy holders, for example, have been used to establish normal values for some tests. However, such individuals are neither a representative sample of the whole population or models for good health. If an individual has a test value outside the normal range, the chances are great that some disorder or disease is present, but test values in the normal range cannot be considered reliable evidence for good health or absence of disease.

Derivation of Optimal Standards

Clearly we need a different set of standards or values as goals for good health. For this purpose we have proposed different standards based on studies of individuals or population groups with maximal stamina and vigor, low incidence of cardiovascular diseases, and exceptionally long, vigorous lifespans. Studies of these individuals have resulted in a series of values that are considerably different from the normal values in common use. Table 1–1 summarizes our current optimal standards and compares them to normal values.

It should be emphasized that the optimal standards are attainable by most people if they are willing to work for these goals, i.e., make the necessary changes in their living habits. Figure 1–1 depicts the broad and continuous range of health-fitness from illness to the optimal range. Techniques for achieving optimal goals or levels are one of the principal features of this book.

Table 1–1

Optimal vs Normal Standards[4]

	Optimal	Normal
Body Weight	Abdominal fat pad: 5–7 mm	Ht.-Wt. table or appearance
Body Fat %	5–10 (to 12 for women)	12–30
Heart Rate (pulse)	<50/min	60–100
Blood Pressure	90/60–120/80	100/70–150/90
Blood:		
Cholesterol	125–175 mg%	150–300 mg%
Triglycerides (fasting)	35–100 mg%	50–200 mg%
Uric Acid	2.5–6.4 mg%	2.5–8.0 mg%
Sugar (fasting)	65–90 mg%	65–110 mg%
O_2 Maximum	38–85 ml/kg/min	20–38 ml/kg/min
Stress EKG	Negative test at 100% max heart rate	Negative test at 75–85% max heart rate
Exercise	30–60 min daily	None to occasional
Diet	Low Fat-cholesterol-salt-protein-sugar	US Diet: High Fat-cholesterol-sugar-salt-protein-calorie
	High Fiber, adequate calcium	Low Fiber and low calcium
Alcohol	0–1 drinks/mo	2–7/wk
Smoking	None	Common
Sleep	7–8 hours regularly	<7, >8 or variable

Optimal Body Weight

The establishment of optimal weight standards is of special importance and deserves more detailed description. Body weight is the simplest, most objective, and accurate measurement that is readily available to everyone. It is a useful indication of general health, endurance fitness, and progress towards optimal health-fitness.

Figure 1–1

Range of Health-Fitness
from Illness to Optimal

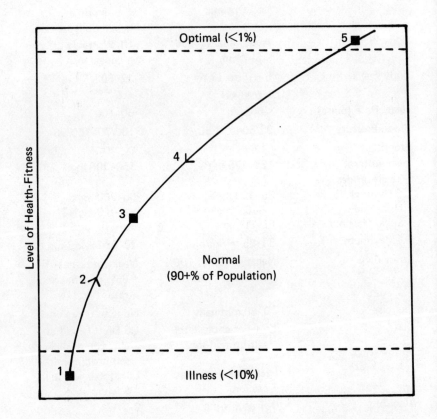

Person No.

1—Has a disabling illness either temporarily or permanently.
2—Is not satisfied with being normal and has changed his living habits from normal to optimal.
3—Maintains a "normal" level of health by following a few fitness practices on a regular basis.
4—Represents a youth or former athlete whose health-fitness is deteriorating.
5—Has achieved optimal health.

People (including physicians) usually decide whether they or others are at "normal" or "desirable" weight by the way they look or feel or by height-weight tables. These methods are misleading because they are not necessarily related to good health, and they do not take into account the large differences among individuals in muscle, bone, fat, and personal bias.

What is needed is a simple, reliable method for determining the optimally healthy weight of each person, regardless of his height, sex, amount of muscle and bone, or observer's opinion. The following method[3] has been tested in thousands of persons over a period of 10 years, and found to satisfy the above criteria.

Measuring body fat. From the standpoint of health-fitness, the important aspect of body weight is the proportion of fat. Excess amounts of fat are closely associated with low levels of physical fitness and high risk for developing such common major diseases as hypertension and diabetes. Therefore, our method focuses on body fat content. The most accurate method of measuring body fat, underwater weighing, is complicated and requires special apparatus not generally available. There is a simpler way that correlates positively with the underwater method. The major storehouse of body fat is directly under the skin, and most of the excess fat is found from the bottom of the rib cage to the mid-thigh. By measuring the amount of fat under the skin near the waistline, one can estimate total body fat. We call this the "pinch test" because skin with fat is pinched between the thumb and forefinger and measured with a caliper.

Optimal body fat. Who should be chosen as models to determine the optimally healthy weight and amount of body fat? Should we measure a large group of so-called "normal" Americans and calculate the average (normal) for them? If we did this, we would be falling into the same trap that the height-weight tables have, i.e., using a population that is known to be overweight, not physically fit, and having a very high incidence of cardiovascular diseases.

On the contrary, it seems logical to us to choose as models of optimal weight and fat a group of people who have the highest level of health-fitness and the lowest incidence of cardiovascular diseases. Fortunately, distance runners fit this criterion and are available at all ages for testing. It has been found that distance runners have body fat measurements of 5 to 10% by the underwater weighing method. Our pinch test of more than 100 men and women distance runners aged 15–70 showed a remarkable similarity in abdominal skin-fold thickness. Their measurements ranged between 5–7 mm (6 mm = ¼ inch) regardless of the height, sex, bone or muscle mass.

Figure 1–2

Optimal Weight Curves
American Women

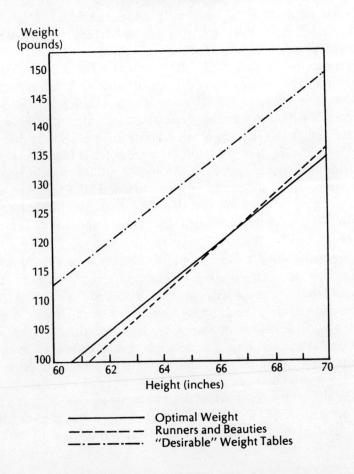

	Optimal Weight
	Runners and Beauties
	"Desirable" Weight Tables

This is the range we use as a criterion for optimal body fat and weight. Abdominal skin-fold thickness measurements were also made on several thousand men and women patients, and volunteers over a period of five years. And 260 of these men and women between the ages of 15 and 89 were found to have a skin-fold measurement equal to that of the distance runners. The height-weight curves of this group were compared with those of the distance runners and a group of 75 national and

Figure 1–3

Optimal Weight Curve
American Men

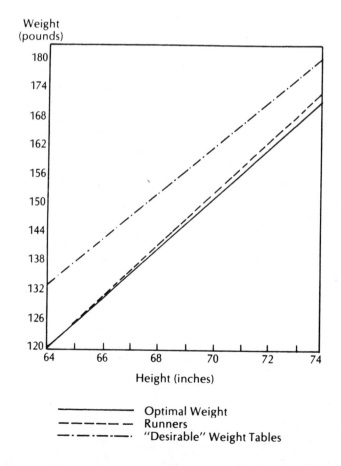

international beauty contest winners. All three groups had similar weights for their respective heights and sexes (Figs. 1–2, 1–3).

A comparison of the data from these three groups with that of desirable height-weight tables commonly in use shows a marked difference: The so-called desirable weights are considerably greater than the optimal weights.

The measurement of abdominal skin-fold thickness is the simplest, most practical way to determine whether an individual is at optimal weight, regardless of body build, age, or sex. With a little practice it is possible to estimate skin-fold thickness yourself without the use of calipers. Determining optimal weight by this technique is more logical, more reliable, and more useful than weight based on normal or desirable height-weight tables or by judging from appearance.

2
Lifestyle
and Longevity

Our concept of optimal health fitness is based on the conviction that the responsibility for personal health rests primarily on the individual. The degree of health and vigor, the avoidance of disease, and the longevity we achieve are almost entirely determined by what we do each day of our lives; i.e., our lifestyle.

Lifestyle

If we practice optimal living habits in daily life, we can achieve the optimal health, vigor, and longevity of our hereditary potential. Failure to do this predisposes us to the diseases that are the major causes of disability and death in the USA: heart attacks, obesity, strokes, high blood pressure, emphysema, diabetes, cirrhosis, some forms of cancer (lung and intestines), and an increased number of accidents.[5] The physician's current function is almost to entirely patch up, alleviate suffering, and take emergency measures associated with diseases that cannot be cured. This amounts to fighting a delaying action in a battle that is already lost. On the other hand, changes in individual living habits before diseases develop may prevent major diseases from occurring.

Now let us examine more closely the relationship between lifestyle and disease. Table 2–1 summarizes typical American living habits—and diseases and symptoms that present scientific information has associated with their abuse. Because diet plays such an essential role in the causation of our major medical problems, it is also discussed extensively in Chapters 9–20.

Longevity

As a person gets older many changes take place in the body and mind. In some, the changes are great and one sees extensive

Table 2–1

Lifestyle and Disease

Living Habits		Associated Diseases or Symptoms
Diet		• Obesity
Excess	Calories, Fat	• Hyperlipoproteinemia
Intake	Cholesterol, Salt,	• Diabetes
	Sugar, Vitamins	• Hypertension
		• Heart Attack
		• Stroke
		• Uremia
Deficiency	Protein	• Cirrhosis
in Intake	Minerals	• Kwashiorkor
	Vitamins	• Osteomalacia, Ricketts
	Fiber	• Osteoporosis
		• Diseases of Intestine: Cancer, Diverticulosis, Functional Disorders
		• Mental Disorder
		• Skin Diseases
Sedentary Life		• Obesity
		• Heart Attack
		• Diabetes
		• Low-level physical fitness
		• Lack of vitality
Smoking		• Cancer (lung, mouth, lips, throat, larynx)
		• Emphysema and Bronchitis
		• Cardiovascular diseases
Alcohol and other Drugs		• Cirrhosis, Heart Disease, Accident Proneness
		• Mental Deterioration, Anxiety-Depression
		• Suicide, Homicide
Attitudes (reactions) toward life situations		• Anxiety-Depression
		• Suicide
		• Psychosomatic Illnesses
		• Unhappiness, Pessimism, Cynicism
		• Lack of Energy, Fatigue

loss of functional capacity; in others the changes are minimal. A few individuals (like Picasso and Michelangelo) remain vigorous both mentally and physically well into their 80s and 90s; others become progressively more feeble in mind and body at a much younger age. So many nursing homes are filled with people in their 60s and 70s who have deteriorated to the mental and physical helplessness that Americans have come to view as inevitable.

What are the characteristic changes that occur with advancing age? Typically we see a progressive increase in body fat accompanied by a loss of muscle and bone mass. We see a gradual decline in physical and mental vigor. In many, blood cholesterol and triglycerides gradually increase. The incidence of high blood pressure, cardiovascular disease, and many forms of cancer increases. Furthermore, these changes are so common in western countries that normal standards have been lowered with advancing age and physicians accept them as the new "normal" range.

For a number of years the Foundation for Optimal Health and Longevity in Bonita, California has engaged in research on why some individuals and population groups are able to maintain vigor of mind and body with advancing age, whereas the majority of individuals follow the course of progressive deterioration cited above. Foundation studies have been done in Ecuador, the Caucuses, Hunzaland, and California. Population groups in Ecuador, Hunza, and the Caucuses were chosen because they have the reputation of being exceptionally long-lived. In Hunzaland and the Caucuses and Equador, documentation was lacking. Nonetheless, it seemed clear to us that there were large numbers of older individuals (over 75) who were exceptionally vigorous of body and mind.

The long-lived people in the three population groups cited above had several characteristics in common:

(1) They engaged in many hours of physical exertion daily, primarily farming, using hand tools. This work involved much up- and downhill walking, and in addition, they frequently carried heavy objects.

(2) The diet was, in general, much lower in calories, protein, animal (saturated) fats, cholesterol, and salt and higher in carbo-

hydrates and fiber than the usual American diet.

(3) They were generally slender, well muscled, and had a vigorous, youthful appearance.

(4) Blood cholesterols (106 to 192 mg%) done on the Ecuadorian group were much lower than the average American of similar age.

(5) High blood pressure and cardiovascular diseases were virtually absent.

Our studies in the San Diego area were done on two groups of individuals: (1) Highly conditioned men between the ages of 15 and 75 who were long-distance runners and who trained and competed regularly over distances of 1 to 26 miles; and (2) a variety of unconditioned, but normal, individuals: schoolgirls and boys aged 9 to 10, individual men and women aged 17 to 69, and firemen and policemen aged 30 to 50. These groups were tested before and after 6 to 12 months of a special exercise and diet program.

The research studies cited above have led us to the following conclusions:

• Daily, prolonged physical activity as a part of an individual's lifestyle is a major factor in the maintenance of physical and mental vigor many years beyond the usual retirement age.

• A diet substantially lower in animal fat, cholesterol, salt, protein, sugar and calories than is present in the typical American diet, is an important factor in the prevention of atherosclerosis (hardening of the arteries) and cardiovascular diseases, and thereby favors an increased life span.

• The older distance runners (California) exhibited physical and blood chemical characteristics similar to those of the long-lived population groups. Furthermore, they maintain high physical and mental vigor, show a low incidence of hypertension and cardiovascular diseases, and have low blood cholesterol and triglycerides. They also resembled the long-lived people in body build.

• Mental and physical deterioration so commonly seen in older individuals in the USA is not part of the normal aging process, and therefore avoidable. Deterioration is due to specific diseases or the result of many years of insufficient use of mental and physical abilities. The principal law of aging is that any function, skill, or tissue that is not used continuously will gradually be lost.

● Properly designed and supervised exercise programs based on endurance activities appear to be equivalent to the physical activities that are a part of the lifestyle of the long-lived population groups. Such programs, combined with optimal diets, have been successfully used by the Foundation on unconditioned individuals aged 9 to 70 to achieve the physical and biochemical characteristics of the long-lived population groups. These programs are applicable to individuals of all ages under the supervision of properly qualified personnel.

● Psychological factors are important for longevity. It was noteworthy that in the long-lived population groups studied there was general expectation of living to 100 or more years. Continuing, useful participation in the social and economic life of the community and the family was the usual custom. Indeed, the very old members of the community enjoyed greater respect and prestige because of the age and experience.

Part Two:
Fitness to Fit You

3
Exercise:
Run for Your Life

- In 1973, Jack Foster, age 42, ran the marathon (26 miles, 385 yards) in 2 hours, 11 minutes, registering the second fastest time in the world for that year.
- In 1975, Dr. Terrence Kavanaugh, a Toronto cardiologist, and six of his postcoronary patients ran the Boston Marathon.
- In 1968, Mary Boitano, age 5, ran her first marathon. At age 10 she ran the fourth fastest women's time in the United States: 3 hours, 1 minute.
- In 1973, Larry Lewis, age 106, was still running 6 miles per day through Golden Gate Park in San Francisco, then working a full shift as a waiter.
- Men, women, children of the Tarahumara tribe in Mexico have a game in which they kick a wooden ball with their feet on a continuous run for 50 to 200 miles.

These people are not biological oddities. In all the animal kingdom, man is the endurance animal, par excellence. Endurance is our natural endowment and a requirement for reaching and maintaining optimal health. Our physical capacities and needs have been shaped throughout millions of years of evolution, yet, in merely a few hundred years, we in the advanced nations have developed a culture that has almost abandoned physical movement. Our symbols of success and leisure are the executive chair and the easy chair. The consequence is an accelerated degeneration of unused muscles and organs—most significantly, the heart.

We can be encouraged, however, because almost everyone, regardless of age or present physical condition, can attain tremendous improvement through a program of regular exercise. As cited above, even those who have had a heart attack may attain a superior level of fitness. Age is no barrier to the determined. At the age of 58, Norman Bright began jogging after 30 years of sedentary living. At age 62 he set 12 world track records for his age group. These anecdotes are cited to emphasize that each of us has remarkable physical capacities of which we are unaware. Even exceptional results require as little as 30 minutes to 1 hour per day, depending on the exercise activity selected.

Exercise improves five physical factors:[6]

- Endurance
- Strength
- Flexibility
- Coordination
- Relaxation

Although all forms of exercise produce some benefit in all five areas, generally one specific form of exercise will emphasize just one. Calisthenics, for example, stretch the muscles and tendons so that the body is flexible in all movements. Weight training (e.g., barbells) emphasizes development of strength; team sports and gymnastics develop coordination. Endurance is improved by activities that challenge the heart and lungs, such as running, swimming, cycling, rowing, rope-skipping, and cross-country skiing.

Aerobic Exercise

A comprehensive program of fitness should include the development of all five factors. But, from the standpoint of optimal health and resistance to disease, we emphasize endurance exercises. These are also referred to as *aerobic exercises* because endurance is a function of the body's ability to deliver oxygen to the muscles and other organs where it is used for producing energy.

The heart, blood vessels, and lungs are involved in this process. The lungs, diaphragm, and rib cage muscles pull in oxygen-rich air and expel carbon dioxide waste. The heart moves this oxygenated blood through 60,000 miles of vessels at up to 40 miles per hour. Oxygen is released to tissue cells from our capillaries (which are in greater number in the physically fit), and our venous system returns blood from our extremities aided by the pumping action of our major leg

muscles. When this system is well developed, we have a trans-
portation network capable of delivering food and oxygen to
nourish the trillions of cells throughout the body.

Training Effect

What exactly is an endurance or aerobic exercise? It is any
activity that is vigorous enough to produce and maintain a heart
rate between 120 and 160 beats per minute depending on age,
conditioning, and other factors.[7] Some authorities[8] state that
the "training effect" (improvement in endurance or stamina)
begins about five minutes after the exercise starts and continues
as long as a heart rate of 120 to 160 (70–85% of maximal heart
rate) is sustained; others believe that it starts earlier.[9]

The most effective aerobic exercises are running, swimming,
and cycling because they achieve the desired heart rate more
quickly and sustain it. Other activities, such as handball, basketball, squash, football, tennis, and downhill skiing, though vigorous, are intermittent rather than sustained. These are more
likely to improve our anaerobic capacity (energy production
without use of oxygen). Such activities, therefore, require
longer periods to achieve the training effect. Activities like
bowling, golf, gardening, calisthenics, and weight training are
usually insufficient to produce the training effect, and therefore, do not develop endurance fitness.

Appendix E compares the energy expenditures of various
common activities and sports. Note the higher caloric expenditures of the endurance exercises.

Physiological Benefits

Heart Rate

After a few months on a physical conditioning program, the
resting heart rate begins to decrease, sometimes quite substantially.[10] It is not uncommon for some who select distance
running as their activity to drop from a resting rate of 70 to 50
and even 40 beats per minute. In a conditioned individual the
lower heart rate indicates that the heart is able to pump more
blood with each stroke and rest more between each beat. Highly
conditioned runners generally have resting heart rates below 50.

Blood Pressure

Exercise can lower blood pressure in many suffering from high blood pressure. Boyer and Kasch studied 23 hypertensive men on a moderate exercise program, consisting of 20 minutes of calisthenics and 30–35 minutes of jogging twice per week.[11] After 6 months, they averaged an 8% reduction in blood pressure. A similar study of 69 hypertensives reported a 6% drop in blood pressure. Hellerstein tested 656 hypertensive men in a somewhat more vigorous program and found an average reduction of 15% in blood pressure.[12]

Collateral Circulation

By "collateral circulation" we mean the increase in vessels serving the heart muscle itself, the coronary arteries. It is a narrowing of a coronary artery that usually triggers the heart attack. The gradual closing off of these vessels causes the heart pain known as *angina* (due to lack of oxygen to the heart muscle). As a result of exercise, blood vessels in all exercised muscles, including the heart muscle, may increase in number and size.[13] If a narrowing occurs in one vessel, other nearby vessels will supply oxygen to the same heart muscle area. This reduces the probability of a heart attack and of death from a heart attack.

In a study by Miller and Galton,[14] 881 heart attack victims were classified according to their pre-attack physical activity. Forty-four percent of the least active group died within 4 weeks of the heart attack; only 20% of the most active group died within this same period. In a similar study of several Israel kibutzes, sedentary workers had an immediate mortality of 23%, the heavy laborers only 5.7%.[15]

Blood Fats

Endurance exercise has been found to lower blood cholesterol and triglycerides (a form of blood fat). Excessive blood levels of these substances are associated with cardiovascular diseases.

Mann conducted diet-exercise studies using medical students.[16] The students were fed a diet high in fats, calories, and cholesterol. He found that as long as the students were physically active, weight was constant and there was no rise in cholesterol or triglycerides. When exercising was stopped, weight, cholesterol, and triglycerides shot up.

Golding exercised 42 men, an hour a day, for nine months. Their average cholesterol dropped from 260 to 195 mg%.[17]

Studies have demonstrated that a high-fat meal raises the level of blood fats by one-third or more, and that this effect usually lasts for 4 to 8 hours. If one exercises after the meal, the fat is cleared from the blood much quicker, that is, it rises less than half as much and disappears more quickly.[18]

Energy Metabolism

Improvement in level of energy is substantiated by both physiological tests and the subjective experience of people. Ability to generate energy can be measured on the treadmill or bicycle ergometer. We see the results of greater energy in improved performance in work and in sports. Fit people demonstrate the ability to work longer, play harder, and endure stress better.

The improvement in capacity for work and play brought about by conditioning results from change in our heart, lungs, blood vessels, blood chemistry, and general musculature. The amount of blood pumped with each heartbeat may double, and flow to the muscles is greatly increased. The overall effect is improvement in our oxygen transport system.

Endurance activity improves the ability of muscle cells to utilize oxygen. Holloszy has shown that long-distance running, for example, may result in a twofold increase in the oxidative enzymes within the muscle cells associated with an increase in the number and size of mitochondria—microscopic particles within each cell responsible for producing the energy the cell needs.[19] At the same time, other enzymes associated with fat metabolism increase, so that the conditioned person is deriving a greater percentage of his general requirements from body fat.

Digestion

The digestive function of the intestines is improved. Exercise stimulates the contractions of the intestines and provides them with better circulation.

Sleep

Studies have shown that we sleep better after exercise.[20]

Physiological studies of changes in sleeping patterns during periods of activity versus periods of inactivity show that, in the active periods, people fall asleep quicker and enjoy a deeper sleep.

Tension

Under tension or stress, chemicals are released to the bloodstream to prepare us for fight or flight. Because our outlets for alleviating stress are usually limited, these chemicals are not used up and may remain in the blood for some time. One such chemical is adrenalin, which increases our blood fats and also the rate of their deposition in the arterial walls.[21] With exercise, we use up these chemicals, especially adrenalin and excess blood fats; with little or no exercise, the chemicals are not used as quickly, leading possibly to harmful consequences. Selye, well known for his research on stress, subjected 20 rats to blinding lights, loud noises, and electric shocks.[22] Ten of these rats who were exercised vigorously, were well and thriving after 10 months. All 10 sedentary rats were dead.

Many of the habits we regard as harmful are forms of escape from the stresses and tensions of ordinary living. Second to life itself, peace of mind may be our highest goal and perhaps the most elusive. We have no formula for perfect tranquility. However, a relaxed mind tends to accompany a relaxed body, and exercise is possibly the most readily learned and most consistently effective route to body relaxation.

Psychological Benefits

The effects of training on the psyche include increased self-confidence, mood elevation, better self-image, ability to tolerate the stresses of daily life, improved ability to relax, and to sleep. Those engaged in a program of regular exercise often overcome living habits such as cigarette smoking, overweight, and alcoholism.[23] This is probably an indirect effect of exercise, i.e., the physically fit individual becomes more self-disciplined and more self-aware.

The effects of conditioning on emotions are largely subjective. However, we are beginning to see objective studies on the effects of conditioning on personality and emotions. Ismail and

Trachtman tested psychological changes in 60 middle-aged men after an intensive four months physical fitness program.[24] They found that the subjects increased significantly in emotional maturity, imagination, guilt proneness, and self-sufficiency.

Appearance

Most of us have friends who have achieved marked improvement in their appearance as a result of programs of physical activity: loss of body fat and improved posture. Bodily beauty and grace of movement are outward manifestations of optimal health. When we say someone looks healthy we mean that he or she appears animated, graceful, and attractive with bright eyes, clear skin, and shapely lithe body. Optimal health-fitness is necessary for attaining true beauty and grace of movement.

Disease Prevention and Longevity

Hammond surveyed 300,000 men over the age of 45 years.[25] He reported that the death rates among those who never exercised were 4 to 5 times higher than among those who exercised a great deal. In a study of 129 heart attack victims, 64 were given a program of exercises for 1 year. In that time, 2 of the exercised patients died and none had angina (chest pain). Among the 65 nonexercised control group, 7 died and 30 had angina.[26]

The majority of Americans die of vascular diseases.[27] Most of the risk factors associated with these diseases are favorably affected by physical activity. Based on 15,000 physical examinations at the Aerobic Center in Texas, Cooper determined that the higher the level of physical conditioning the lower the blood pressure, blood lipids, body fat, EKG abnormalities, etc.

The key question about the effect of physical conditioning on aging is whether it can slow the rate of deterioration of function. Dehn and Bruce analyzed 3 longitudinal studies (studies that extend over years) on the effects of physical conditioning. They found that the rate of decrease in cardiovascular function was 2 times faster in the inactive than in the active.[28]

In Finland, long-distance skiing is a lifetime activity. Karvonen compared the survival of Finnish champion skiers to that

of the general Finnish male population.[29] In the general Finnish
male population 50% were still alive at age 65, whereas among
the skiers 50% were still alive at age 72. It was interesting to
note that at age 90 more than 10% of the skiers were still alive
compared to 2% of the general male population. Similar indirect
evidence of the beneficial effects of regular physical activity is
available from many other sources.[30]

Lessons from the Tarahumara

The *Tarahumara* (meaning foot runner) are a cave-dwelling
people who live in the rugged Sierra Madre Mountains of northern Mexico in the state of Chihuahua. About 50,000 of them
live widely scattered in about 26,000 square miles of rugged
mountains and deep canyons with virtually no contact with
other people.

They are famous for their extraordinary endurance; the
ability to run for one to three days continually, day and night,
over rugged terrain at high altitudes. This is done as a game
(called *rarahipa*), a traditional activity in the lifestyle of these
remarkable people.

We were members of an expedition composed of physicians,
exercise physiologists, nutritionists, distance runners, and pho-
tographers sponsored by The Foundation for Optimal Health
and Longevity. In May 1974, we visited a Tarahumara village to
study their lifestyle and to make physiological measurements
pertaining to their running ability. We came away from our visit
even more impressed with the extraordinary ability of the
Tarahumara than we were from reading about them.

Rarahipa is played by men, women, or children in teams. Betting of cloth, livestock, money, and blankets is an important
feature of the races. Each team has a solid wooden ball about
three inches in diameter, hand-carved from the balled root of a
juniper or madrona tree. We witnessed two such races: one for
women and one for men, and were astounded by their performance. They ran 50 and 60 miles, respectively, over hilly, rocky
terrain, almost entirely in the darkness of the night. They pro-
pelled the wooden ball, on the run, with a flick of the foot,
while wearing thin-soled sandals.

Our studies reveal that the runners were similar physically and in blood chemistry to long distance runners that we had studied previously in California. They were small, at optimal weight, well-muscled, had low to normal blood pressures, and slow resting pulses. Their blood cholesterols and triglycerides were optimal, and their blood sugars showed no evidence of diabetes.

The diet of the Tarahumara consists primarily of corn and beans, with only occasional milk, eggs, meat, and fruit. Their total caloric intake appeared to be approximately 1500 calories per day.

Our studies led to the following conclusions:

• The Tarahumara are capable of repeated feats of extraordinary endurance under extremely difficult conditions (of terrain, altitude, and darkness), living on a diet far below our standards of adequacy in protein, calories, vitamins, etc. Clearly, our beliefs and concepts on nutrition for the athlete, as well as the average person, needs to be reexamined in the light of these observations. The findings are in keeping with our studies showing that diets much lower in calories, fat, salt, and cholesterol than are contained in the typical American diet are adequate for very active people. They also conform to our belief that extra vitamins are not necessary for extraordinary physical exertion, and, therefore, not needed by the average person.

• The Tarahumara are capable of extraordinary feats of physical stamina without formal training. It emphasized the enormous training value of daily physical exertion (walking and running) from early childhood. This occurs naturally in a culture devoid of vehicles, situated in a rough mountain terrain, with individuals living widely scattered, and having a traditional activity demanding superlative endurance. This combination of circumstances has apparently resulted in an ideal endurance training program.

How can we duplicate these conditions in our society, which has made it progressively more difficult to obtain physical exertion in daily living? There are several approaches: (1) endurance activities as part of the physical education program in the elementary schools, (2) courses in optimal health-fitness in the schools and colleges, and (3) the introduction of a 30- to 60-minute period of physical exertion in our daily life.

The absence of diabetes in the Tarahumara examined by us suggests that diabetes is uncommon in these people. This is noteworthy because a tribe related in origins, the Pima Indians of Arizona, who are sedentary and tend to be obese, have been found to have the highest incidence of diabetes in the world (49% of adults). This suggests that daily living habits are capable of overcoming a strong genetic abnormality.

4
Definition of Physical Fitness

There are a variety of ways to define physical fitness. Some authorities believe a simple, yet comprehensive method is to use five factors (endurance, flexibility, strength, coordination, and relaxation) as the basic criteria. Use of this method allows for each factor to be evaluated and also improved with proper training.

Each of these five factors makes an important contribution to your total physical fitness, and there is an essential interrelationship between all five. This is especially true in terms of achieving optimal health-fitness. We believe that two factors (endurance and flexibility) should be given the highest priority in the achievement and maintenance of optimal health-fitness.

Endurance Is the Best Insurance

Endurance is the ability or capacity to do continuous physical work. It relates closely to the health and vigor of the cardiovascular-respiratory system (heart, blood vessels, and lungs) and can be described as the ability of the body to take in and use oxygen for the performance of physical work. The type of physical activity that develops endurance is large muscle (legs, arms, and trunk) action of a continuous nature performed at below maximal intensity.

It is important to distinguish between *aerobic* and *anaerobic* activity. Aerobic exercises (which increase endurance) must be performed at a low enough level of effort to allow the body to take in and use oxygen equal to the demands of the activity in which the individual is engaged and not incur an oxygen debt. This kind of exercise challenges the cardio-respiratory (heart-lung) system, which responds by gradual improvements in its capacity (adaption). In contrast, anaerobic exercises (used to increase speed and strength) are performed close to maximum effort, and leave one breathless in a short period of time because the body's demand for oxygen exceeds the ability of the cardio-respiratory system to take in oxygen and deliver it to the active muscles.

To judge the type of activity in which you are engaged, see how long you can continue it before you must stop and "catch your breath." If you must stop frequently (every few minutes) to recover, it is mainly an anaerobic activity. If you can continue for 15 to 30 minutes, it is largely an aerobic activity.

Examples of endurance activities are walking-jogging-running, swimming, cycling, rowing and cross-country skiing. These activities develop a progressively higher level of heart-lung fitness. Because walking-jogging-running requires few learned skills, a minimum of equipment, expense, and instruction, can be practiced alone or in groups, and is the most efficient conditioning method, it is the "exercise of choice."

Flex-Time

Flexibility is of greater significance to long-range health than many people realize. Like endurance, it may be gained or lost every day of one's life, depending on our proper attention to it. Flexibility may be defined as "joint mobility" or "range of motion" of joints. A *joint* is where two bones contact, end to end. There are many kinds of joints in the body, but the ones we are primarily concerned with are called diarthrodial or "freely moving joints." These joints are surrounded by a fibrous sac, which is filled with a lubricating fluid (synovial fluid).

The structures of the joints that hold the bones together, yet permit various degrees of movement, are called ligaments. *Ligaments* are tough, fibrous bands that attach bone-to-bone. Another structure crossing the joint is the tendon. *Tendons,* fibrous extensions of muscle, pull on the adjacent bone when a muscle contracts, thus causing movement. A third joint structure is *ligamentous fascia*—the key to flexibility. This fascia forms a sheath around muscles that shortens and becomes stiff after a period of inactivity. We may, for example, be unable to straighten an elbow after it has been in a cast for a few weeks. Over a long period of inactivity, this shortening contracture affects our posture, as illustrated by the bent-over position of most old people in our culture. This peculiar characteristic of fascia, is a gradual, continuous, and almost imperceptible shortening. It is a prime cause of injury, post-injury disability, and the posture and movement limitations of the aged. Prevention is accomplished by moving the joints through their complete range of motion on a daily basis. (A program for optimal flexibility is described in Chapter 7). Certain joints seem to be more susceptible to tightening: the ankle, knee, hip and lower back.

Ankle Flexibility. Ankle joint range of motion should be between 80 and 90 degrees to be considered optimal. Besides being a hedge against tendonitis, flexible ankles allow the body's center of gravity to tip forward easily, thus allowing the forward movement that is part of all running activities.

Flexible ankles also provide a better base of support in squatting and lifting activities, allowing the large muscles of the thighs and hips to produce the power for lifting rather than the weaker muscles of the low back. The greater the mobility of the ankle joint, the less chance there is for tendonitis and later rupture of the Achilles tendon, a common problem of inadequately trained individuals in some aerobic programs.

Knee Flexibility. Knee joint flexibility is closely related to hip and low back stability. The muscles that flex the knee also extend the hip, so they involve two joints. All running activities require movements at these joints. The length and effort required in each stride is based on the flexibility of the knee and hip. Flexibility of the knee involves muscles that flex the hip (forward movement of the leg as in kicking).

We'll consider hip extension first. The hamstring muscles (back of upper leg) extend the hip and flex the knee. The consequences of tight hamstrings—pulled muscles, early fatigue, increased energy consumption, and shortened stride—are frequently underestimated. Inadequate range of motion at the knee contributes to a tight Achilles. Tight Achilles also transmits greater pressure to the ball of the foot with resultant excessive stress on bones and ligaments between the ball of the foot and the heel (arch). **2050124**

Hip Flexibility. Tight hip flexors (muscles that lift the thigh) probably have more adverse effects on both daily living and athletic performance than any other flexibility problem. They frequently contribute to chronic low back pain. The primary hip flexors have attachments on the front of the lumbar vertebrae (lowest five vertebrae) and on the front of the pelvis. If they shorten, through failure to perform stretching exercises, the pelvis rotates forward causing a permanent malalignment in the spine (sway back or lordosis).

In athletic performance the flexibility of the hip joint relates directly to freedom of forward and lateral movement. During the running stride, any limitation of hip extension (by tight hip flexors) reduces the stride length, and therefore speed and efficiency.

Low Back Flexibility. Low back flexibility (ability to bend forward easily at the waist) is essential to good posture, general body health, and the body mechanics required in sports. The movements of this joint are controlled by abdominal muscles, back muscles, and the hip flexors and extensors referred to above. If tight hip flexors are combined with weak abdominal muscles, lordosis (excessive sway back) and low back pain is the likely result. Once we have achieved optimal flexibility, continued stretching of tight muscles and strengthening of opposing muscle groups is necessary to maintain proper balance. An inflexible lower back can cause considerable pain and disability, a very common problem in adult Americans.

Strength for Length

Strength is the ability to exert force. The muscles and joints of the human body are not built for great strength. Rather, they are designed for range of motion, coordination, and speed. A wiry arm may be capable of throwing a baseball much faster than a brawny one. The majority of our tasks in both athletics and daily life are accomplished more through coordination than brute strength.

From the standpoint of optimal health-fitness, optimal strength is a matter of one's ability to move one's own body weight with efficiency and agility in a variety of situations. This does not require bulging muscles nor hours of weight training.

Abdominal. Abdominal muscle strength affects posture and is essential for effective action of both the upper and lower extremities. Next in importance are the hip and knee extensors (muscles that enable us to rise from a squatting position). However, it is difficult to separate these two groups functionally because they work together during walking, running, and jumping activities. Other areas where optimal strength is important are elbow flexors and extensors, shoulder area, hand (grip) and toe muscles.

It is important to recognize the close relationship between flexibility, strength, and posture. The movement of each joint involves opposing muscles. To flex (bend) a joint, we must also be able to extend (straighten) it. These opposing forces (muscles) must be in balance. This can be illustrated by imagining a telephone pole held upright by guy wires. If the wire on one side is pulled tighter (is stronger) than the opposing side, the pole will lean. The body is balanced like a pole, with muscles and ligamentous structures holding the segments in proper balance. If either tightness or weakness occurs, a variety of problems may result.

We have mentioned that weak abdominal muscles and tight low back structures are a primary cause of many low back problems. A solution to these problems is to strengthen the abdominals and stretch the low back. We should also use our strong hip and knee extensors for heavy lifting rather than imposing excessive strain on the relatively weaker back musculature. Abdominal muscles support respiration, such as forceful exhalation during vigorous exercise. The attachments of the abdominal muscles to the rib cage support throwing, hitting, and pushing movements carried out primarily by the muscles of the shoulders and arms.

The value of strength in the upper extremities is apt to be less evident. We recognize it mainly in emergencies when we are faced with the need to lift a fallen person, hold on to a ledge until help arrives, or climb out a window during a fire.

Our toes are weak due to our practice of wearing hardsoled shoes and walking on smooth surfaces. This behavior pattern contributes to the gradual weakening of the small muscles of the foot. Optimal strength in these muscles is needed for healthy feet, and provides adequate force for running activities.

Coordinate Your Skills

Coordination is the ability to carry out a variety of movements smoothly and efficiently with a minimum of unnecessary
action. It may be an inherited characteristic. However, it is difficult to identify general coordination as a distinct ability and
most research suggests that coordination ability may be specific
to a given activity.

Coordination relates to the development of specific skills
and timing which is crucial to the progressive mastery of skills.
Optimal nervous patterns, which must be established before
coordination is achieved, are a function of special brain cells
located in the cerebellum. General exercises for improving
coordination will be presented in chapter 9.

Endurance is affected by good coordination because the
"synchronization" of arm and leg movements eliminates
unnecessary effort and reduces fatigue. Coordination also deter-
mines our effective strength. Strength is a combination of the
number of muscle fibers, their size, and the coordinated contraction of these fibers.

Relax, Relax

Relaxation is the opposite of tension, a state of low muscle
stimulation. At night, during sleep, the body renews itself. For
those untrained in the techniques of relaxation, sleep is perhaps
the closest they come to experiencing deep muscle relaxation,
yet deep muscle relaxation can be learned and experienced in
the conscious state.

It may help to understand deep muscle relaxation by thinking
of the muscles as being in one of three states:

(1) *Totally relaxed* (little or no recordable electrical activity).
This is complete muscle rest and a state the muscle can maintain
for relatively long periods.

(2) *Tonus:* characterized by muscle readiness and measurable
electrical activity. The muscle in this state is ready to do something. Many people spend most of their waking hours in this
state. Because each muscle in our body has a counter-muscle to
pull in the opposite direction, a great deal of energy can be

wasted in this tense state. People who remain continuously in the state, usually feel fatigued much of the day.

(3) *Fully contracted:* characterized by a hard, firm muscle generating a great deal of electrical activity. It is impossible to hold a muscle in this state very long, due to the build-up of waste products of muscle activity. Continued full contraction without a resting phase can even result in pain, trembling, and numbness. Most of us have experienced this pain when carrying a heavy suitcase over some distance.

The ability to voluntarily relax the entire body allows our muscles to recover from the tensions of daily living. Only when the body has the capacity to rest and recover can training for optimal fitness be successful. During periods of strenuous activity, in work, recreation or athletics, muscle relaxation is vital to conserve energy. In our culture daily life offers few opportunities to discharge this muscular tension and as a consequence many of us feel chronically fatigued. Yet relaxation is a skill that can be learned through proper exercises. Several of these exercises are described in Chapter 22.

5
Your Health-
Fitness Profile

Before undertaking an exercise program designed to achieve optimal health-fitness, you should have a special type of examination. We call this the Health-Fitness Profile. Ideally, everyone should have the complete profile, but unfortunately most physicians are not equipped for this extensive an exam.

Individuals under the age of 30 who have been exercising regularly and are free of disease by the usual medical examination, may begin their program without certain parts of the profile. We strongly recommend the complete profile in those over the age of 30, especially those who have not been engaged regularly in vigorous physical activity.

The purpose of the profile is threefold:

● To detect diseases (primarily cardio-vascular-pulmonary and musculo-skeletal disorders) that would prevent daily vigorous physical exertion.

● To assess the degree of risk for a heart attack (coronary risk factors).

● To determine the initial level of health-fitness so that an appropriate conditioning program can be designed for each individual.

● To evaluate progress.

Chart 5–1 is used as the record for this series of examinations. Note the focus on health rather than disease. This means special emphasis on nutrition, physical activities, and coronary risk factors, which are not a part of the conventional medical examination. Conventional tests such as chest x-ray, complete blood count, and urinalysis should be done before the Health-Fitness Profile. Blood chemistries including cholesterol, triglycerides, uric acid, and glucose on a blood specimen are part of the profile. The special tests include a maximal-stress EKG test on the treadmill by the Bruce Method, measurement of the percent of

body fat by the skinfold thickness method, and calculation of
maximal oxygen consumption using the Astrand-Rhyming test
on the bicycle ergometer. Two running tests, the 1-mile run and
the 12-minute run are also administered.[31-35]

When the Health-Fitness Profile is completed, the individual's
level of Health-Fitness may be calculated by our numerical
rating system (the E-C System—see Chart 5–2). Note that each
factor or measurement (18 in all) that has an influence on
health and fitness is assigned a numerical rating from +10
to −10.

Most of the units used in the system are self-explanatory, but
a few need clarification. The "heredity" ratings are based on
correlations between some diseases (hypertension, diabetes,
obesity, heart disease) and family history, i.e., the fewer of
these in your family, the better your chances are of not getting
them. The "personality" category refers to the theory that
personality type is important in heart attacks. Type A, for
example, hard-driving, tense, is very susceptible to heart
attacks.[36]

The highest possible total score is 135 for men and 140 for
women. Individual ratings range from Optimal to Below Normal
(very risky):

E-C Rating	*E-C Score*
Optimal	over 100
Above Average	over 60
Average or Normal (risky)	40–60
Below Normal (very risky)	below 40

Chart 5-1

NAME	ADDRESS				PHONE	AGE	BIRTHDATE
PRIVATE PHYSICIAN	ADDRESS			REST			

DIET

MEALS	SNACKS	EGGS	MEAT	MILK	CHEESE	VEG.	FRUIT	COFFEE	SWEETS	ICE CREAM	SALT	MISC.
D	D	WK	D	D	WK	D	D	D	D	D	D	

PHYSICAL EXERTION

HIGH SCHOOL	POST GRADUATE	PRESENT (past 2 years)

SMOKING

PACK/YEARS	ALCOHOL	TYPE	AMOUNT	FREQUENCY

WEIGHT

16-20 YEARS	PAST YEAR	MIN.	MAX.	REMARKS

DISEASES

H.B.P.	DIABETES	C.V.D.	JOINTS	SURGERY	INJURY	REMARKS

MEDICATION

PAST	PRESENT

FAMILY HISTORY

	H.D.	AGE	DIABETES	H.B.P.	OBESITY	REMARKS
FATHER						
MOTHER						
OTHER						

PHYSICAL EXAM.

HT.	WT.	REST PULSE	EST. OPT. WT.	POSTURE: KYPHOSIS LORDOSIS FEET	DATE
MUSCLES	ARMS	ABDOMEN	LEGS	HEART: SIZE SOUNDS	
TONE				LUNGS	FUNDI	PULSES

ESTIMATED POTENTIAL	REMARKS

DATA SHEET	DATE			
MVO$_2$ (TREADMILL)				
MVO$_2$ (BICYCLE)				
ONE MI. RUN (TIME)				
TWO MI. RUN				
THREE MI. RUN				
TWELVE MIN RUN (DISTANCE)				
BODY FAT % — ABDOMINAL				
BODY FAT % — O-SITE				
BLOOD STUDIES — CHOLESTEROL				
BLOOD STUDIES — TRIGLYCERIDES				
BLOOD STUDIES — URIC ACID				
FLEXIBILITY — ANKLES				
FLEXIBILITY — HIP/KNEE				
FLEXIBILITY — BACK				
STRENGTH — ABDOMEN				
STRENGTH — UPPER				
STRENGTH — LOWER				
COORDINATION — UPPER				
COORDINATION — LOWER				
COORDINATION — GENERAL				
RELAXATION — GENERAL				
RELAXATION — SPECIFIC				
WEIGHT/R.P.R.				
BLOOD PRESSURE				
GOALS	5 MILE			

1 HOUR				10 MILE			

Chart 5-2
E-C System
Health-Fitness Rating

POINTS	10	7.5	5	2.5	0	-5	-10
B.P.	90-110/50-70	111-120/71-80		121-130/81-85	131-139/85-89	140-160/90-100	>160-100
CHOL. (mg%)	125-175	176-200		201-225	226-275	276-350	>350
SMOKING	Never		Ex-smoker 1 yr. or more		>3/d	4-20/d	>20/d
DIABETES	FBS<90 2 hr.<100	no diabetes	Diabetes optimal Control		Diabetes Fair control		Diabetes Poor control
T.G. (mg%)		<100		<150	150-199	200-300	>300
EXERCISE	Optimal 30-60 min. daily		Regular but not optimal		Occassional	None	
DIET	Optimal	1	2	3	4	5	U S Diet*
ALCOHOL		0-1 mon.	0	1	<7/wk	>7/wk	Alcoholism
HEREDITY			0	1	2	3	HD Obesity HBP Diabetes
PERSONALITY			Type B		AB Mixture	Type A	
EKG			Normal		1	2	3
URIC ACID (mg%)			<6.5		<8	>8	
BODY FAT	5-10%		<15%		Male<20% Female<24%	Male >20% Female >24%	
PULSE (resting)	<50	<60		<70	<80	>85	
02 MAX ml/kg/min	>60	>52	>42	>34	>28	<28	
SLEEP			Regularly 7-8 hrs.				
SEX			Women <50 yrs.				
AGE			<30	30-50	51-69	>70	

*Excessive cholesterol, fat, sugar, calories, salt, and protein; too little fiber.

6
One-Two-Three, Testing

For the best possible program of optimal physical fitness, it is necessary to measure the initial status of fitness as well as the changes that occur during the progress toward the goals. This chapter describes some practical methods for doing this.

Endurance

Fitness testing for endurance usually require tests of maximal cardiovascular-pulmonary capacity or function. Ideally, this should be done only on individuals who have passed a complete medical examination that includes a maximal stress EKG test, for example, the Health-Fitness Profile (Chapter 5). Those who are under the age of 30, or who have engaged in maximal physical exercise on a regular basis for years, may forego the stress test, though we recommend it for everyone as good insurance against unexpected cardiac or pulmonary difficulties. In any case, a physician or other health professional who has experience in cardiopulmonary resuscitation should be present during the testing for maximal physical capacity.

Bicycle Ergometer Test (Astrand-Rhyming)

This test employs a special stationary bicycle (e.g., the Monarch Ergometer), which has an adjustable and precise work load.[37] The change in heart rate each minute over a period of 6 minutes is recorded at an appropriate work load for each individual. Maximal oxygen uptake (VO_2 max), which is the best measure of endurance fitness, is estimated from the heart rate obtained during 6 minutes of pedaling at a constant rate (50 pedal turns per minute). (See Appendix D.) The principal advantage of this test is its safety. The subject is seated, under close surveillance, and makes only a submaximal effort.

Other advantages of the test are its simplicity, the elimination of motivation as a variable, its short duration, the minimal equipment necessary, good reproducibility, and satisfactory correlation with other methods.

Twelve-Minute Run Test

This test is simple to perform and requires no special equipment or assitance. It is best done on a standard quarter-mile track, which is found at high schools and colleges. If none is available, a suitable distance can be measured on a level country road or field, using a car or bicycle odometer. It may also be performed indoors on a measured track or floor. Running or gym clothes should be used.

Because the test is for maximal physical capacity, the subject should cover as much distance as possible up to the point of near-exhaustion. He or she may, of course, stop, walk, jog, or run, depending on the level of fitness and ability. The exact distance covered in 12 minutes is recorded, and the level of fitness and maximal oxygen consumption found in Table 6–1.

Mile-Run Test

This test is similar to the 12-minute run test except that the person being tested covers exactly 1 mile at his maximum speed. The time this takes is the measure of his endurance fitness. This test should be done on a standard 440-yard track for accuracy. It has the advantage of being easier to record results than the 12-minute run, especially when a group of individuals are being tested simultaneously. Table 6–2 gives the relationship between the mile time and VO_2 max.

Heart Rate

One of the best measurements of your body's reaction to physical exertion is the heart rate. It can be counted manually as a beat at the wrist (radial artery) or under the jaw (carotid artery). By counting your pulse immediately upon awakening in the morning, you can establish a base from which to evaluate your progress. This is your resting heart rate. Resting heart rates between 60 and 100 per minute are considered normal.

Table 6–1

Classification of
Cardiovascular-Pulmonary Fitness
(Adapted from the Cooper 12-minute test)[41]

Grade	Distance (miles) covered in 12 minutes	Maximal O_2 consumption ml/kg/min
I. **Very poor:** Patients with cardiovascular-pulmonary diseases, marked obesity, musculoskeletal diseases.	<0.5	<24
II. **Poor:** No disease, but markedly impaired cardiovascular-pulmonary fitness, obesity.	0.5–1.0	24–28
III. **Borderline:** The "weekend" athlete.	1.0–1.24	28.1–34
IV. **Fair:** Those engaged in nonendurance sports on a fairly regular basis and the ex-athlete.	1.25–1.49	34.1–42
V. **Good:** The level reached by many after 3–10 months of a good endurance exercise program. The recommended goal for most people.	1.50–1.74	42.1–52
VI. **Very Good:** The level achieved by a minority after a year or more of a good endurance exercise program. Recommended level for the competitive athlete (nonendurance sports).	1.75–2.0	52.1–60
VII. **Superlative:** The competition endurance athlete.	>2.0	>60

Table 6–2
Cardiopulmonary Fitness
Related to Mile Run Time

Mile time (minutes)	Approximate Maximal O_2 consumption (ml/kg/min.)
12:00	27
11:00	30
10:00	33
9:00	35
8:00	38
7:00	44
6:30	48
6:00	53

Those who develop high levels of endurance fitness often have resting heart rates below 50 per minute. The resting pulse rate gradually goes down over a period of months of regular endurance training. It is useful to keep a record of your resting pulse rate so you can follow the process of cardiovascular adaptation to optimal physical fitness training.

Another test of endurance fitness using the heart rate is the rate of recovery of the heart rate following maximal physical exertion. A heart rate below 100 per minute, 1 to 2 minutes after maximal exertion indicates optimal endurance fitness.

Multistage Treadmill Test (Bruce Method)[39]

This test is used primarily to determine whether an individual has coronary heart disease and to observe whether disorders of the rhythm of the heart occur with exercise. It can also be used to estimate maximal oxygen consumption if it is continued to the subject's maximal level of exertion. In this respect, it is the safest of all of the tests because it is done with constant EKG surveillance, with a trained physician and resuscitation equipment at hand throughout the test.

The test is started at a treadmill speed of 1.7 miles per hour and a slope (incline) of 10 degrees. Every 3 minutes the speed and grade are increased according to a special protocol until the subject cannot continue any longer, or some symptoms occur that require terminating the test. The test protocol is shown in Appendix D. The disadvantages of this test are the need for expensive equipment, highly skilled personnel, and long duration, as compared with the other tests.

Flexibility

Joint flexibility is relatively easy to measure and is specific for each joint. Although everyone develops a general lack of joint flexibility due to years of inactivity, each individual has particular joints that are "tighter" than others. Thus, a person may have loose upper extremities, but be very tight in the joints of the lower extremities. The classic test of flexibility is the "toe toucher (A)." Bend forward from the waist with feet together and knees locked; try to touch the ground with the finger tips. A very flexible person can place his palms flat on the ground, while one with inflexible joints may have difficulty reaching past his knees.

There are four areas which must be stretched regularly if one is to attain optimal flexibility of the lower half of the body: (1) the back of the ankle, or Achilles areas, (2) the back of the knee, or the hamstring area, (3) the front of the hip, or hip flexor areas; and (4) the low back area. Some simple means of measuring joint mobility are as follows.

Ankle (Achilles tendon). Stand barefoot with feet together, facing a wall (B). Place the toes against the wall and bend at the knees. The knees should touch the wall easily without the

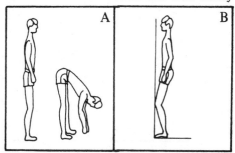

heels being raised from the floor. Now move your toes away from the wall at least 2 inches. Repeat the action. If your knees can again touch the wall without raising the heels from the floor, you have a reasonable degree of ankle flexibility. If you can accomplish the same task with toes 3 inches from the wall, you have adequate flexibility. Success at 4 inches indicates an optimal degree of ankle flexibility.

Knee (hamstrings). Stand on a step with feet together and knees locked in a straight position on steps with toes even with the front edge (C). Bend forward at the waist and reach downward with the hands toward the toes. You should be able to touch the top of your arch without undue strain. If you can touch your toes or the level of the step on which you are standing, your knee flexibility can be considered adequate. The ability to reach beyond the step level at least 4 inches indicates optimal hamstring flexibility.

Hip. Lie on your back on a bench or table with your hips near the end (D). Grasp the right knee with both hands, and pull it slowly toward your chest, allowing the opposite leg to relax or hang over the table edge. Bring the right knee as close as possible toward the shoulder. This tests the left hip flexors for flexibility and if your left leg comes up above the horizontal, you have considerable tightness in the area. If the left leg remains horizontal during the pulling of the right knee, you have reasonable flexibility. If the left leg remains hanging below the table level, then you can be assured of having optimal flexibility in the anterior hip area. Repeat the test for the opposite hip by bringing the left knee toward the shoulder.

Low Back. There are a number of positions in which the flexibility of the low back area may be tested. However, it is some-

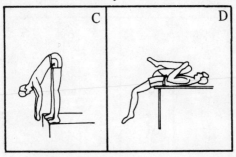

times difficult to differentiate between tight hamstrings and a tight low back. A large amount of ligamentous fascia in the low back area makes it prone to inflexibility for most people in industrialized societies because the sedentary life rarely requires stretching of this area of the body. The first step is to kneel on the ground sitting on your heels. Bend the trunk forward as far as possible, resting the buttocks on your heels (E). You should have no trouble laying your head on the ground in front of your knees unless your low back is extremely tight. The next step is to sit on the ground with legs straight and feet about 3 feet apart. Now bend the head and shoulders toward the right knee, then the left (F). If you can touch your forehead to each knee, your back and hamstring flexibility can be considered optimal.

A second test can be done by assuming a sitting position on the ground with legs straight in front and feet together. Place an eight-inch book between the knees and bend the head forward until the forehead touches the book. If you succeed, you have optimal low back and hamstring flexibility. Finally, you can isolate the low back component of flexibility by lying on your back with hands resting on both knees. Gradually pull the knees toward their respective shoulders until the tightness in the low back prevents movement (G). If you can touch both knees to the shoulders at the same time, you have optimal low back flexibility.

Strength

There are several areas of the body where optimal strength is especially important. Methods of testing yourself in these areas are described below.

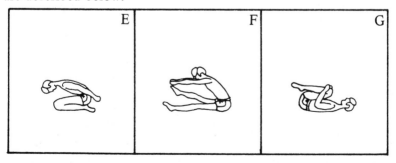

Abdominal

Strong abdominals are an aid to good respiration and a major hedge against the common "low back syndrome." There are several ways by which the strength of the abdominal muscles can be tested. Start in the most basic position of lying on the back with knees bent and feet flat on the ground (H). In this position, slide one hand under the small of your back to become aware of the spinal curvature in this area. Now tighten the abdominal muscles until you flatten the spinal curve to the ground. Hold this position and slowly slide one foot away from the buttocks and straighten the knee, always keeping the back flat with abdominal tension. Next, slide the other foot downward so that both legs are straight and resting on the ground. If you can maintain this flat back position for 30 seconds with legs straight, you have passed the first test of abdominal muscle strength.

Now assume the beginning position described above. Raise the arms and reach toward the knees, raise the chin to the chest, now raise the shoulders and upper back off the ground as you reach toward the knees with the hands, hold a partial "sit-up" position for 20 seconds, and you have passed phase two. The classic bent-knee sit-up is both a test and an exercise for abdominal muscle strength. Repeat the partial sit-up exercise 10 to 20 times, resting between "holds" before progressing to the final test of abdominal strength. When you are able to complete 50 consecutive bent-knee sit-ups, you have achieved optimal abdominal muscle strength.

Knee and Hip Extensors

Strong knee and hip extensors give a good base for all lifting activities and save frequent injury to smaller low back muscula-

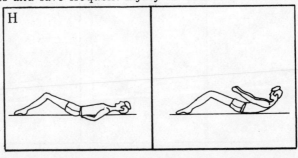

ture. The strength of the knee and hip extensors is evaluated by two methods: (1) direct measurement of force exerted against a dynamometer or cable tensiometer, and (2) a determination of the amount of weight pushed or lifted. The basic aim of optimal strength fitness is to be able to handle your own body weight efficiently. Therefore, it is not necessary to have elaborate apparatus to determine the adequacy of your knee and hip muscles. The simple knee bend (partial squat) requires good strength in both these areas, and when you are able to complete 25 partial knee bends, your muscles in this area may be considered in good shape. The knee bend should be stopped when the lower leg is at a right angle to the thigh in order to avoid injury to the knee joint. Doing the complete knee bend has no advantage, and may cause knee joint injury if done repeatedly. Optimal leg strength can best be determined by the number of single leg "dips" you can do. When you can complete 10 dips on each leg (holding onto an immovable object for stability), you have achieved optimal strength in this area.

Upper Extremities

There are three primary areas of the upper extremities where optimal strength is important. The best test for the *elbow flexor group* is the simple "chin-up" with palms away from the face on a horizontal bar (I). The first level test is to hold the elbows at right angles while grasping the bar and maintain this position for at least 10 seconds. The next test is done by hanging from the horizontal bar and bring the chin to the bar at least 10 times. The accomplishment of this task indicates you have optimal elbow flexor strength. The *elbow extensor group* can best be tested by some form of the "push-up" exercise. Assume a prone position on the ground with hands placed beside the shoulders

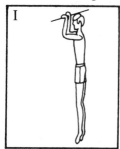

I

and toes in contact with supporting surface, keep the knees and
hips in a straight line, and extend (straighten) the arms until
they are perpendicular to the ground (J). Now, with only the
hands touching the ground, repeat the up and down exercise
30 times in succession, and you will have achieved the optimal
performance for this area of strength. Another means of measuring this area is on the parallel bars (K). The exercise is called
"dips" and is begun by supporting the body by the hands from
the two bars in an erect position. Then gradually lower the
shoulders toward the hands and return to the starting position.
Completing this activity at least 10 times indicates optimal
strength performance.

In order to evaluate *grip strength* properly, a small hand dynamometer is necessary. A grip strength (in pounds of force) of
150 pounds for the dominant hand of men and 85 pounds for
women can be considered optimal. The nondominant hand
should be not less than 90% of the dominant one.

Lower Extremities

The strength of the muscles in the feet and toes is often
neglected with adverse effects on both lower extremity health
and maximal athletic performance. An exercise that strengthens
this area can also test whether your feet and toes have optimal
strength. Place an object weighing about 3 pounds on one end
of a bath towel lying spread out on the floor (L). Then, with
the heel of the tested foot held firmly on the floor at the end
opposite from the weight, grasp the towel with the toes, and
pull firmly inward and toward the body. Do this as fast as
possible, repeatedly grabbing, pulling, releasing, and regrabbing
the towel with the toes. If you are able to pull the weight on
the towel to the stationary foot within 10 seconds, you have
optimal strength in the feet and toes.

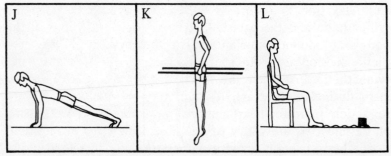

Coordination

Measurement of coordination is usually tested by performance in a game or contest involving special skill and techniques. The ability of body parts to work together as a smooth functioning unit depends primarily on practice—thousands of repetitions done correctly. We refer you to books written about your specific sports interest (tennis, racquetball, etc.), appropriate tests of coordination in the specific skills.

Unfortunately, scientific research has not yet established a reliable test for general coordination or neuromuscular skill. Balance, reaction time, eye-hand coordination, and adaptation of all these systems to specific skills are involved. Several approaches to this category of fitness testing are described by Cureton: The Balance Beam Tests and The Figure Eight Agility Run.[40]

Relaxation

Our bodies function in a dynamic balance between muscle activity and relaxation. Relaxation is difficult to measure, but degree of muscle tension can be measured quite accurately by means of an electromyograph. This machine is capable of detecting tiny action potentials (electrical currents) from the contracting muscles and recording the level in microvolts on graph paper or some other form of visual readout. What is measured is not relaxation directly, but rather the reduction of electrical activity. The same is true of other ways of evaluating relaxation.

The dynamic balance between physical activity (tension) and relaxation is a shift in our nervous sytems between the sympathetic and the parasympathetic systems, divisions of the body's autonomic (involuntary) nervous system. The sympathetic division tends to speed up bodily processes; the parasympathetic slows them down. The sympathetic system is dominant during physical activity and stress—it prepares the body for action. Increased heart and breathing rates, as well as tensing of the muscles, are a few of the observable signs of increased sympathetic nervous activity. Other signs are increased blood pressure, elevation of the level of sugar in the blood, and redistribution of blood supply to increase the blood flow in the muscles.

Because the signs of sympathetic nervous system activity are more observable or detectable than those of the parasympathetic system, we test for relaxation by measuring the decrease of sympathetic nervous activity. By establishing base lines for pulse rate, respiration, and general muscle tension, we can monitor relaxation by observing their increase or decrease.

Other observations that can be used to estimate the degree of relaxation are: (1) resistance to passive movement of a limb (arm or leg), (2) irregularity and force of respiration, (3) abdominal vs. chest breathing, (4) involuntary movements or contractions (e.g., blinking), (5) sudden, involuntary jerks or movements, (6) speed of responses, (7) appearance of tension around the eyes and face, and (8) muscle tone.

7
Basic Program of Optimal Fitness

Principles of Optimal Health

The objective of optimal exercise is for you to achieve your maximum potential of physical fitness. This level varies widely from individual to individual, but is predictable with considerable accuracy by analysis of the health-fitness profile (Chapter 5). It depends largely on age, genetic endowment, and previous physical training.

Individuals with no obvious disease (the *apparently* healthy), who are unconditioned (untrained), generally have a maximal oxygen consumption ranging from 20 to 38 milliliters of oxygen per kilogram of body weight per minute. Experience indicates that it is possible to condition these individuals up to levels of 38 to 85 ml/kg/min (optimal fitness levels). Conventional conditioning methods are designed to improve—not to optimalize—physical fitness. This is a much more limited goal, which can be achieved in many ways and without the special coaching and techniques necessary for achieving optimal physical fitness.

Ideally, physical exertion should be a daily habit, built into the daily living pattern just like eating, sleeping, and working. Unfortunately, modern society has virtually eliminated all jobs that require enough cardiovascular exertion to achieve optimal fitness levels. For this reason, individuals in our society must schedule a daily period for such exertion.

Walking-Jogging-Running

What type of activity is most effective to achieve optimal fitness? It should be one that increases the heart rate to a certain level (70 to 85% of the maximal level) and maintains this level continuously for a period of at least 30 to 60 minutes. Walking-jogging-running is the quickest, simplest, most efficient, and least expensive method for accomplishing this objective. It has the additional advantages of requiring no special skills, equipment, or facility. It can be done alone or in groups, anytime of day, anywhere, indoors or out. It exercises most of the muscles of the body as well as the heart, lungs, and blood vessels, and is suitable for lifelong use. It gives you the opportunity to be alone with your thoughts or together with family or friends. It is, therefore, the basic activity for achieving optimal fitness or your best performance in any sport.

Other forms of physical exertion (tennis, skiing, cycling, etc.) serve in a secondary capacity: for variety, fun, improving coordination, flexibility, strength, relaxation, and agility, or as a substitute when injuries prevent walking or running. These are recommended as weekly or biweekly activities to supplement the basic conditioning of the walking-running program. To achieve optimal levels of physical fitness using other forms of endurance activity requires longer periods of training than 30 to 60 minutes per day.

If you have not engaged in physical activity for many years (and especially if over 60 years old), or have a very low level of fitness (less than an O_2 max. of 24 ml/kg/min, and or are more than 35 pounds over optimal weight, you should begin with 15 minutes per day (1% of the 24-hour day). Most others can safely begin with 30 minutes per day of walking. Thirty to 60 minutes per day is the minimal time needed for achieving optimal fitness.

The intensity of the exertion is most simply measured by the pulse rate. Everyone should learn to count their pulse during exercise (you may stop briefly to do this) to control the intensity of the exercise and to measure recovery rate following exercise. The goal is to maintain a pulse rate of 70 to 85% of one's individual maximum pulse rate. In most individuals this means 22 to 28 beats every 10 seconds. Optimal recovery is achieved when pulse rate is 16 or less beats every 10 seconds, 1 to 2 minutes after terminating exercise at the intensity described above.

The warm-up and the warm-down are essential parts of the conditioning process and should not be neglected because of disinclination or lack of time. See below.

Variety and attractive surroundings contribute significantly to making the exercise program enjoyable and maintaining the motivation for the lifelong habit pattern of daily physical exertion. We recommend that you find a number of different places to do walking-jogging-running with an eye to natural beauty and convenience: parks, open countryside, etc.

It is important to develop good posture and style while walking and running to encourage muscle relaxation, maximal breathing capacity, and to minimize muscle-tendon-joint injuries. Every effort should be made to practice good form during the daily exercise period after the defects in style have been identified.

During the course of your daily routine there are many opportunities for obtaining additional physical conditioning exercise. For example, walking to and from your car, climbing stairs, walking to lunch, doing calisthenics while dressing in the morning, and isometrics while riding in a vehicle.

The two most practical times to do your concentrated period of exertion are before breakfast and before dinner. Other people find lunchtime fits into their daily routine well.

To continue any activity for a lifetime requires strong motivation and continuing enjoyment. Competition can be a strong motivating force, a pleasurable social occasion and a source of exciting satisfaction. Running provides an endless source of self-competition, and in many areas, opportunities for peer competition in all age groups and at all levels of proficiency. Bettering your time for any given distance or competing with your peers are powerful motivating forces and the source of continuing satisfaction once you have reached a certain level of physical fitness. For most individuals this level of fitness is reached after about 6 months of conditioning.

Reaching optimal physical fitness requires 12–18 months of an optimal conditioning program for most unconditioned individuals.

Warm-Up!

The warm-up may be described as physical activities engaged in before vigorous physical activity with the purpose of:

- Preparing the physiological systems of the body.
- Preparing the psychological systems of the body, and
- Reducing the probability of musclotendon-joint injuries.

There are numerous examples of instinctive preparation for action in the animal world. The stretching movements of members of the cat family after sleep is a good example. Even humans, when awakened from a sound sleep, often arch their backs, straighten their legs, and reach out with their arms to overcome the stiffness that accumulates during inactivity.

Singers warm-up by practicing a series of progressive vocal exercises before their performance. Automobile engines perform more efficiently after a few minutes of idling.

The warm-up stretches the connective tissue to maintain flexibility. Beneath the skin is a thin layer or sheath called "ligamentous fascia" (see Chapter 5). It covers the muscles and keeps them from "popping out." Around the joints this sheath often thickens to provide additional stability and prevents dislocations. Unfortunately, it tends to shorten with the passage of time, and this shortening process is slow but constant. Every day this fascia shrinks unless opposed by specific exercises to stretch it. Ballet exercises are the best example of the form of warm-up that stretches and maintains flexibility of the ligamentous fascia.

The warm-up shifts blood to the active muscles. An active organ requires a large blood flow to fulfill its greater need for oxygen and nourishment. When muscles are inactive, there is very little blood flow to and within them. During vigorous physical activity the oxygen requirement of muscles may increase as much as 25 times. To accomplish this requires a shift of blood to the exercising muscles. This is best accomplished by a proper warm-up period. A study by Barnard showed that strenuous exercise without proper warm-up resulted in abnormal EKG findings, which were eliminated by preliminary jogging of from 2 to 5 minutes.[42] Warm-up not only increases circulation but also increases the mobility of the joints.

Warm-up activities may be divided into two types, general and specific. Both are useful for preparing you effectively for maximal physical exertion. General warm-up involves large muscle movements not related to a specific activity or sport. Jogging before a tennis match might well come under this heading, as would "jumping jacks" before a football game; in other words, actions that raise the body metabolic rate but are not part of the activity itself.

Specific warm-up exercises involve actions that are part of the activity being prepared for: practicing strokes with a tennis racquet, shooting baskets with a basketball, and playing catch before the baseball game would all be classified as specific warm-ups. Others are: taking starts from blocks (sprinting), swinging a bat (baseball), playing catch (baseball or football), shooting baskets (basketball), high kicking (high jump), short sprints (basketball or football), hitting tennis balls against a wall (tennis), trunk-twisting (discus throwing), or knee lifts (running).

An Enduring Plan

In earlier chapters we have described the principles of an optimal exercise program and the benefits that accrue from it. The purpose of this chapter is to present the basic program of activities that will help you attain your own optimal level of physical fitness.

Major emphasis is placed on endurance activities because they form the base of the total optimal health-fitness program. The first few months of your program will be primarily endurance oriented, supplemented with daily flexibility exercises. After a few months of concentration on these activities, the other three factors of physical fitness are added to the weekly program. At the end of this chapter a program grid is presented as an aid to the development of your optimal fitness.

Let's say your health-fitness profile (Chapter 5) has just been completed and analyzed. It shows that you have no disease (of heart, lungs, joints, or muscles) preventing you from doing vigorous physical exercise daily. In addition, it indicates that your level of physical fitness (as measured by the maximum oxygen uptake) is in the usual but unconditioned range (20–38 milliliters of oxygen per kilogram of body weight per minute). An optimal diet has been prescribed to start you toward your optimal weight and optimal blood chemistries (cholesterol, triglycerides, glucose, and uric acid).

Walking-Jogging-Running

One endurance exercise has many advantages for those who persevere beyond the first few months it takes to reach an adequate level of fitness. Actually it is a set of related aerobic exercises that are among our most natural activities: walking, jogging, or running.

They are the most economical of all sports or recreational activities, require the least equipment, least expense, and least time. They may be done alone or with companions, at any time of day or night, on city streets, parks, mountain trails, or ocean beaches. They are inborn capabilities requiring no learned skills, and they can be enjoyed by either sex and at any age from one to 100. They enable you to explore your own community and other towns and cities at a pace that allows you to become intimately acquainted with the surroundings. They provide an escape from the cares and concerns of the day, an opportunity to meditate without fear of disturbance, or simply to commune with nature.

You have a clear-cut choice to satisfy your competitive instinct, to challenge only yourself, or to relax and walk or run as you wish. Experienced runners report pleasant, long-lasting euphoria and sense of well-being, which appear to be the consequence of the prolonged and rhythmic movements of the entire body.

Equipment. Before starting your program we suggest you purchase a few basic items:

(1) A small diary or log book to record your daily activities: type of exercise, duration or distance covered, and your reaction to each session. This will help motivate you to maintain regularity as well as provide a record of your progress.

(2) For walking-jogging-running proper footwear is essential. The design and structure of the training shoe should provide plenty of room for the toes (more square than pointed), fit snugly around the heel with a firm (rigid) heel counter, and have thick soles of rubber for the entire length of the sole with

at least ½-inch thickness under a wide heel.[43] Thin seamless socks of stretch material are preferable to avoid blisters and overheating of the feet.

(3) Loose fitting nylon running shorts, T-shirt or sleeveless shirt of perforated nylon, and a cotton or nylon sweat suit complete your outfit. You may need to protect vulnerable areas of the feet from excessive friction with vasoline or tape.

Site. Choose a site for training that is convenient and pleasant. If a standard 440-yard track is available, take advantage of it. Later, when you have developed more endurance and a sense of pace, you will find that a variety of surfaces and areas for your training will lend spice to the daily running sessions. Parks, golf courses, backyards, and back streets are all potential running courses that can be measured and marked to fit your needs. Any place you feel comfortable while running that is not dangerous because of traffic, animals, or terrain is satisfactory. Use smooth-surfaced level areas until your endurance and muscle-tendon-joint strength have reached fairly high levels (6 months or more). The key to developing a healthy heart-lung system is the duration and regularity of the activity. It is important, therefore, to emphasize from the beginning that "how far and how long" you go in your daily exercise routine is far more important than "how hard and how fast." A brisk 2-mile walk is much better than a 440-yard sprint.

Technique. Depending on your maximal oxygen uptake and your previous exercise experience, you should start walking from 15 to 30 minutes daily. Your walking speed should be regulated by your pulse rate (heart rate per minute), which may be measured at the wrist (radial pulse), in the neck (carotid pulse), or directly over the left chest wall (direct heartbeat). The objective is to achieve a pulse rate of from 22 to 28 beats per 10 seconds.[44] To obtain the rate per minute, multiply the number of beats in 10 seconds by 6. Your first goal is to be able to walk 30 minutes nonstop maintaining a pulse rate of between 22 and 28 beats per ten-second interval. The second goal is to be able to walk 2 miles in 29 minutes or less. When you achieve the second goal, you are ready to begin jogging (arbitrarily defined as a pace of 8 to 11 minutes per mile), provided you have reduced your weight to less than 35 pounds over the optimal level.

The art of running, itself, is simple if one relaxes and doesn't try to "run like someone once told me to run." Preconceived concepts on form will probably cause more problems than any other factor. Jogging and running are merely extensions of walking, and are accomplished most efficiently with an upright body (erect posture), arms bent at the elbows between 80 and 120 degrees. (If relaxed, the arms will swing loosely at the sides and slightly across the body in opposition to the leg action.) The hands should cup slightly, and the head should be held high, balanced evenly at the top of the spine. Deviation from the erect posture is apt to cause excessive muscle tightness, fatigue, and decreased efficiency of movement.[45]

Begin with a short, almost shuffling gait (stride) with toes pointing forward and striking the ground with the heel first. Do not try to run on the toes or balls of the feet because this causes too much strain on the muscles of the calves and the Achilles tendons (heel cord). Your initial walking-jogging program should be a 5-minute walk followed by five minutes of stretching exercises as described in Chapter 7 under "Flexibility." This is the warm-up period. Then begin very slowly and continue the jog for 50 yards or so (about 50 steps) slowing gradually to a walk, and then walking about 50 yards. Then repeat an easy jog another 50 yards. After about ¼ mile, or four jogging sets, stop and count your pulse rate. If it is above 28 beats per 10 seconds, continue to walk until it returns to about 20 beats per 10 seconds, before starting the alternating walk-jog routine again. Continue this pattern for 15 to 20 minutes, then finish off with about 5 minutes of walking and stretching.

Don't overdo the first few days of the program. Keep the reins in check, be satisfied with being out in the fresh air and actually beginning a new way of life. Many people with good intentions never really get into a running program because they try to do too much too soon, and develop excessive fatigue or painful muscles and joints. Gradually over a period of weeks you will reach your next goal: continuous jogging for 20 minutes at the target heart rate (22–28/10 seconds). As the body slowly adapts to the imposed demands, increase the jogging portion of your exercise to 110 yards with a 55-yard walk. Later, jog a full lap (440 yards) before walking and so on to the steady slow jog of 20 minutes. About this time you will be ready to take two tests (1 mile for time and the 12-minute run), which are described in Chapter 7. These tests should be repeated periodically every 4 to 8 weeks, to measure your improvement in physical fitness.

The next step is to increase gradually the duration of your daily workout up to 30 minutes by jogging slowly for 4 to 5 minutes followed by stretching (the warm-up period), and then increasing to a speed which you can maintain comfortably for 20 to 25 minutes.

One day per week you should do a longer workout beginning with 31 minutes and gradually over a period of several months increase it to 1 hour. These longer sessions are best done on weekends or holidays in your favorite or most attractive area when you are well rested. This type of run is often made more enjoyable if it is done with friends who are at your level of fitness, or perhaps slightly more advanced. Be cautious in trying to increase your mileage too quickly. Be certain that your body has adapted to one level of fitness before moving on to the next higher level or challenge. Adaptation to each level usually takes 2 or 3 weeks or longer.

Some of the goals you will be working toward during the second 6 months of your training program are: a one-mile time of less than 7 minutes; a 2-mile time of less than 15 minutes; a 3-mile time of less than 24 minutes; and a continuous jog of 10 miles. Our experience over the past 10 years indicates that these goals are realistic ones for well-motivated individuals of both sexes aged 10 to 60 years.

It should be emphasized, however, that these goals were achieved by individuals who followed the outlined programs under the supervision of qualified instructors; during weekly coaching sessions progress was evaluated, and weekly assignments were given based on *individual progress.*

Keep in mind that everyone from the beginner to the Olympic champion needs expert coaching to achieve his (her) personal optimal level of performance. The speed with which these goals are reached depends on age, natural ability, and dedication, but the majority of individuals we have coached have achieved these goals in about 1 year.

After about 6 months of training, when some of the goals have been achieved, you may be ready to enjoy the thrills of

competing in "fun runs." We have found that for most people
peer competition in low-key races is a powerful motivating
force toward the achievement of optimal fitness and the satisfaction and joy that accompanies competition.

A Flexible Plan

Flexibility exercises, commonly called "stretching," must be
done every day for optimal results. The program is geared to
take each joint through its complete range of motion (ROM) as
frequently as possible. Each individual's joints vary considerably
in what may be considered normal ROM; however, average
ROM's for most joints will be found in Appendix D. Flexibility
is limited by joint structure, the length of ligaments, fascial
rigidity, and muscle extensibility. Flexibility exercises and
endurance activities are the two factors that must be included in
each training session.[46]

Warm-Up

Although many people like to begin their training sessions
with stretching exercises, we suggest a period of relaxation and
slow jogging (enough to raise a light sweat) for about 5 minutes
before beginning flexibility exercises. Preliminary jogging
improves circulation and the ability of the muscles to lengthen
and shorten, while decreasing their resistance to movement.
This will not only help you do a better job in your exercises,
but will decrease the chances of muscle-tendon-joint injuries,
which can occur from hurried or strenuous stretching of "cold"
muscles and tendons.

Stretching

When you finish a short warm-up jog, find a grassy area to do
the following flexibility routine. With feet spread slightly more
than shoulder-width apart, begin with a gentle trunk-revolving
movement: easy movements at first to one side and then to the
other, gradually increasing the arc until you can rotate your
shoulders to at least a right angle to the front-facing hips (A).
After 10 repetitions of the trunk-twister you are ready to work
on other joints. The time spent in this phase will depend on the

stiffness or flexibility of the individual (10 to 20 minutes is a reasonable time range if carried out daily).

Ankle. The testing procedures described in Chapter 6 can also be used to improve ankle flexibility. An effective way to increase the flexibility of the posterior area of the ankle is to place one or both feet three to five feet away from a wall, place hands on the wall while supporting the body, and lean forward gradually (B). If you keep the knee locked straight and the heels firmly on the ground as you continue to lean forward, you will feel tightness or strain in the Achilles tendon and in the hamstring muscles. This means that you are stretching the correct structures. Hold this position to the count of ten, then stand erect and relax. Repeat this exercise several times, gradually placing the toes further from the supporting structure, to the point of discomfort.

Another method of stretching the posterior ankle area (tendons, muscles, and fascia) is to stand feet together, with the balls of the feet supported on the edge of a step or curb. Hold on to a rigid object to steady yourself. Then let the heels drop below the curb level as far as possible, and hold this position to the count of twenty. Then step off the curb and rest and repeat this stretching action several times.

Knee (hamstrings). Because the muscles that flex the knee also extend (straighten) the hip, positions that place both ends of the muscle-tendon complex under tension (stretch) will be most effective in achieving optimal flexibility. The sitting position, which our body assumes many hours daily, is a major factor in the tightness of the hamstrings. The first step in stretching the hamstrings is to stand, feet widespread, gently allowing the trunk to fall forward toward one leg and then the other. Repeat this at least five times with each foot gradually

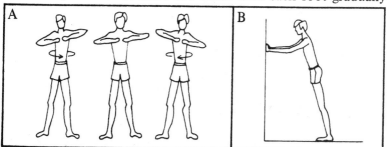

bringing your head closer to the knee and foot on each side. You will feel a pulling sensation behind the knees if you're doing the exercise properly. Next, take a sitting position on the ground with one leg extended straight in front and the other leg bent with the foot brought up close to the hip. This is called the *Hurdler's position* (C). With the left leg extended to the front, support yourself with the left hand and reach forward with the right hand toward the left toe. Lean your trunk on the left thigh, and try to keep the left knee flat on the ground. This will prove difficult at first, but with daily practice your hip and knee flexibility will show marked improvement. After about 10 seconds in this position, relax, and reverse leg positions. Spend several minutes alternating leg positions, each time pushing a little harder toward the restriction, stopping at the point of pain. Unless the joint is regularly taken beyond the usual range, improved flexibility will be slow to develop.

Another effective method for increasing the flexibility of the hamstrings is twisting stretch exercise. From a standing position with the right leg crossed in front of the left, place the left hand on the right shoulder (D). Bend the right arm at the elbow and as the trunk bends forward, twist to the right. Drive the right elbow backward and upward to help the twist. Repeat this twisting and relaxing activity 6 times before switching legs and hands and repeating with the opposite limbs. This exercise can best be accomplished by a gentle and progressive bouncing movement, attempting to get the head closer to the knee with each action.

Low back. The low back area is the natural curve in the lower spine just before the spine meets the pelvis. It is well protected with a massive build-up of ligamentous fascia and is therefore prone to tightness. There are several precautions that should be

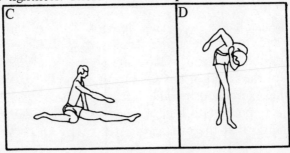

taken to prevent undue tightening in the lower back. They are involved with proper sitting, standing, sleeping, carrying, and running postures.

Begin your back stretching exercises by assuming a position lying on the back (supine) with both knees bent to about a 90-degree angle. Grasp one knee with both hands and pull it toward the chest, at the same time sliding the opposite foot downward until the knee is straight (E). Hold this position until the count of ten and then let the knee down to a resting position with both feet on the floor before repeating the exercise with the opposite leg. If this movement can be accomplished easily, take the same beginning position on the back with the knees bent and feet flat on the ground. Grasp both knees with the hands and pull gently toward the chest holding the maximum position with each knee close to the corresponding shoulder for 10 seconds. Then repeat five times. Each repetition should bring an increase in the range of motion with the goal being to touch each knee to the corresponding shoulder and then raise the head up between the knees and hold for 10 seconds.

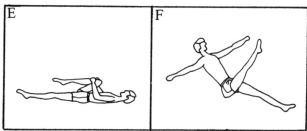

Another exercise that increases the flexibility of the lower back is one similar to the twisting exercise described under knee flexibility. It is begun by taking a spread eagle position on the ground (lying on the back) with arms spread perpendicular to the trunk and hands held palm down to the ground (F). Flex the hip and twist the lower trunk so that the right foot approaches the left hand by crossing the body. Remain in this position for the count of ten and return to the starting position. Repeat the exercise using the left foot, and repeat each six times. It is important to hold the arms and upper back flat on the ground so that the primary stretch occurs in the low back area.

From a standing position, a good exercise is to flex the right knee and grasp it with both hands (G). Pull vigorously toward the chest while balancing on the left foot. Repeat this with the left knee, and each time pull the arms a little harder. Six repetitions can increase low-back flexibility temporarily and be effective as part of the warm-up for vigorous exercise.

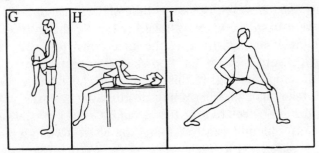

Hip flexibility. These exercises are aimed primarily at the anterior (front) structures that help to lift the knee. The first exercise starts from the position described in Chapter 6 for hip flexion testing. Lie on your back with the hips just on the edge of a table or bench (H). Grasp the right knee with both hands and pull the knee toward the chest allowing the left leg to dangle over the edge. Hold this position for 60 seconds and then repeat with the opposite leg. To increase the stretching action of the anterior hip in this position, two modifications are helpful:

(1) Have a partner hold the thigh of the dangling leg horizontal while you pull upward on the other knee toward the chest.

(2) Tie a weight to the hanging foot and remain in this position for 5 minutes. Attempt to relax the hanging leg as much as possible and then change the weight to the opposite foot and assume the same actions.

In the front lunge position (I), place the hand on the back of the hip near the joint of the leg which is to the rear. Move the weight (body) forward on the bent front leg, and at the same time press downward with the hand on the hip. The front of the hip thus juts forward and is in an excellent position for maximal stretching on one side. Then change the lead leg and repeat with the other hip. Do at least six repetitions with gentle bouncing movements, alternating from one side to the other.

Stronger, Sharper, More Relaxed

Strength, coordination, and relaxation, which supplement the basic fitness factors of endurance and flexibility, will help you increase the enjoyment and effectiveness of your health-fitness program. However, it is not mandatory to include these three factors in your daily program. Suggestions for their inclusion in a weekly training program can be found on the Training Grid at the end of this chapter.

Strength

Optimal strength is concerned with your ability to handle your own body weight effectively in a variety of everyday situations. The kind of work that you do, your recreational pursuits, personal and other factors should be considered before deciding what optimal strength should be. The "overload principle" is the key to successful strength development. Briefly, the concept holds that to increase the strength of any muscle group it must be required to do more than its usual task.[47] Progressive resistance exercises lend themselves well to the kind of strength desirable for the majority of health-fitness conscious people.[48]

Abdominal Musculature. The abdominal muscles are perhaps most important for optimal strength. The first step is to be aware of them and of their role in good posture and in stabilizing the pelvis as a foundation for leg movements. When the abdominal muscles contract, the abdominal wall is pulled inward (toward the spine), the natural curve of the low back is flattened (less concavity), and the front of the pelvis is tilted upward.

There are several positions in which a person can do abdominal exercises. In a sitting position, pull in the abdominal wall and hold for 10 seconds, then relax; repeat ten times. In a reclining position with the knees bent and feet flat on the floor, tighten the abdominals until the low back is flat on the floor ... hold there for 10 seconds and relax, then repeat ten times. Assume a standing position with the back against a wall, feet about two feet out, and knees and hips slightly bent (J). Now tighten the abdominal wall until the low back is flat against the wall ... now slowly straighten the knees and hips (sliding the body up the wall) and move the feet closer to the wall—all the time holding the entire back flat against the wall. Maintain this position for 10 to 15 seconds before relaxing and then repeat five times.

The above exercises will get you started on the road to a firm, strong abdominal wall, which will contribute greatly to your health and performance. Further progress can best be handled by a series of progressively more dfificult exercises, which are begun from the standard sit-up position (lying on the back with knees and hips bent, feet flat on the floor).

After having successfully accomplished the "back-flattening" exercises without strain or discomfort, you advance to the next step, which is to raise the shoulders and upper trunk off the floor, while reaching the hands toward the knees—hold this position for the count of ten—then slowly lower the trunk and head to the floor and relax. Repeat this exercise at least ten times.

The second stage is to perform a sit-up (curl the chin to the chest and slowly bring the trunk upright) touching the forehead to the knees (feet held down or under a rigid support) and then return slowly to the starting position on the floor; relax, take a half breath, hold, then repeat the movement. Gradually you will progress from 10 to 50 consecutive sit-ups at each session. You will benefit by doing a set of abdominal exercises both in the morning and evening.

The next level is to use gravity as the resistance in your routines by performing the exercises on an "incline-plane" (head lower than the hips) (K). With hands held either on the abdomen or behind the head, gradually increase the number of sit-ups you can do until you reach fifty. Progressively heavier weights can be placed behind the neck to achieve higher levels of abdominal strength.

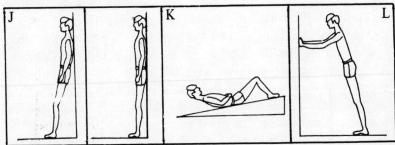

Hip and knee. To improve these muscles, some preliminary work should be done. Brisk walking, over varied terrain, is an excellent way of getting the legs ready for more strenuous strength-building activities (cover the two miles in 30 to 40 minutes).

Phase two is stair climbing. Locate a flight of stairs at least 20 feet high with a fairly steep incline (30–40 degrees). Walk up the stairs (two at a time if small) with a steady rhythm, emphasizing the straightening part of each stride (lifting the body weight). Relax during the walking down and keep a hand on the side rail. Once you have accomplished 8 to 10 repetitions of this exercise, increase the work load on the muscles involved by taking three or four steps with each stride.

Next, progress to running up stairs, 5 to 10 times (depending upon the length and intensity of the effort).

The final step in the hip-knee development is weight training, with the weights (barbell) held on the shoulders and ½ squats done. Three sets of 3–5 repetitions each will result in a high degree of strength development for the lower extremities.

Upper body. Weakness in this area is common in our society, but super-strength in this area is not necessary for optimal fitness. Unless your livelihood or sport demands exceptional strength, the ability to handle your own body weight in hang and support positions, and easily manipulate the implements or equipment of a game are adequate optimal strength.

Modifications of "push-ups and pull-ups" are excellent for strength development of the upper extremities. For the elbow extensor group (triceps), begin with the simple exercise of leaning against a wall with your hands, feet placed from 3 to 4 feet away; push the body away to arms length and return with nose close to the wall (L, M). Be able to repeat from 20 to 30 times before moving to the next step in the progression.

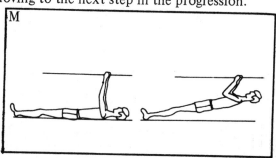

Placing a greater proportion of the body weight on the hands, rather than the feet is a method of increasing resistance and thus strength. Begin by moving the feet further away from the supporting surface, and progress to the standard horizontal push-up position. Using weights (bench press, military press and single arm dumbbell presses) for progressive resistance is the ultimate stage of strength development for this muscle group.

The elbow flexors (biceps) are not as easy to develop progressively (using your body weight as resistance). However, the same principle as used with the push-ups can be applied.

Begin by lying on the back and extending the arms perpendicularly to grasp any horizontal surface or bar at arms length. With the heels remaining in contact with the floor, pull the body up as far as possible by flexing the arms, then allow the body to return slowly to the reclining position; repeat from 20 to 30 times before attempting the next level of pull-ups on a regular horizontal bar.

The accompanying diagrams will show smaller increments in the progression routine. If you are unable to complete one standard "chin-up" you should begin by holding a "flexed elbow hang" for about 10 seconds and repeat from 5 to 10 times. The standard "chin-up" is excellent for developing optimal upper body strength. Two arm curls with a barbell, beginning with about one-quarter of your body weight, is one gradual way of developing elbow flexor strength. Three sets of 10 repetitions, 3 times per week, will result in rapid progress. Gradually work towards a goal of handling half your body weight in two arm curls.

Virtually all exercises that require you to hold onto a weight or surface will result in the development of grip strength. Supplemental programs can be added such as squeezing a tennis ball, and rolling the barbell down to the tips of the fingers and returning from 6 to 10 times.

Coordination

Most of the training to develop optimal coordination should be done in the context of the sport or activity that you enjoy doing (tennis, raquetball, baseball, basketball, etc.). *Timing and balance* are two important aspects of general coordination, so that any activity providing practice in these areas will be valuable.

● Rope-skipping and Aerobic dancing (a system of vigorous, prolonged dancing developed by Sorenson) are both excellent for optimal levels of coordination and endurance.

● A good upper body coordination exercise can be done in an eight-count rhythm by extending the arms from side to hands on chest, front to chest, side to chest, and overhead to chest, repeat gradually increasing the pace (N).

● Similar patterns using hopping (first to the side and then front and back rhythms following a six-count beat) are helpful for the lower extremity coordination.

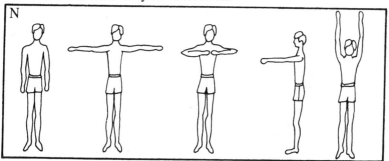

Relaxation

Although relaxation is one of the five factors of physical fitness, it has broader implications for optimal health. A program for improving your ability to relax cannot adequately be described here and is best learned under the supervision of a qualified instructor. Kraus has developed a simple series of exercises to help the individual achieve more from his vigorous activities:

(1) Lie on back, with knees flexed.

(2) Close eyes and take a deep breath, inhale deeply and exhale, rest.

(3) Inhale, rest.

(4) Pull up shoulders to ears and let go. Repeat and let go.

(5) Drop head to the left and then to the right, then to the left and then to the right.

(6) Raise forearms from elbow and drop them.

(7) Drop one leg and bring it back, drop the other leg and bring it back, inhale deeply, exhale.[48]

Try this series of relaxation exercises from 5 to 10 minutes each day before you begin your jogging and stretching routine. Additional relaxation methods are described in Chapter 22.

Warm-Down!

Although the subject of warming down has not had as much attention as the warm-up, it is equally important. It restores normal resting body conditions more quickly, and counteracts nausea, headache, muscle cramping, and helps to eliminate waste products (metabolites) that have accumulated during the activity. Such metabolites (e.g., lactic acid) can result in discomfort and soreness of the muscles for hours or days.

The warm-down is a gradual reduction of effort that allows the body systems to shift gradually to a lower level of physical demand. The greater the intensity of the activity, the longer and more gradual should be the warm-down activities.

Immediately after vigorous or maximal effort, shoes should be removed, loosened, or changed and sweat clothes put on. Light jogging, interspersed with periods of walking, periodic rest, and stretching of areas especially taxed during the effort should then be done. These should be continued until breathing returns to normal, sweating ceases, and the pulse rate returns to within 20 beats per minute of the resting rate.

The alternate contracting and relaxing of the large muscles of the lower extremities during the warm-down period act as a pump to aid in the return of the blood to the heart, and thus maintain a high flow of blood through the exercised areas. This speeds the replenishment of oxygen and nutrients, and the removal of waste products during the recovery period.

Tune to Your Program

It is not possible to recommend a training program that will fit the needs of all, or even a majority of, individuals. Because of the extreme variation in initial fitness levels, potential fitness capacity, differing rates of progress, age, sex, preference for physical activities, and dedication between individuals, it is an unwise procedure to have a fixed schedule for all. These variations emphasize the need for expert guidance (coaching) along the path toward optimal health-fitness. The expert coach can size up the above factors for each individual and design an appropriate starting program. He can then make the proper changes at regular (weekly) intervals, based on the individual's response to the training schedule and his progress in the training program. This is the best way of making steady progress toward optimal goals and for protection against injuries, early plateauing, discouragement, and drop-out.

How To Use the Grid

The following pages contain sample programs at different stages of conditioning based on our experience with large samples of unconditioned individuals of both sexes, aged 10 to 60 years. Note the application of our philosophy—emphasizing endurance and flexibility activities during the first few months of the program. After you have developed a minimal base of conditioning in these two factors, you can begin to vary, substitute, and enlarge on the fitness activities you enjoy with better assurance of continued progress toward the goals.

By spending 30 minutes per day, you are investing 2% of your day to improving the quality of your life, decreasing the risk of cardiovascular diseases, and increasing the probability of vigorous longevity. Now refer to Sample Program 1. Follow the numbers for one day of the week; for example, Tuesday: (1) easy jog for 3 minutes, (2) stretching exercises for 10 minutes, (3) walk and jog for 12 minutes, (4) more gentle stretching for 5 minutes, followed by, (5) 10 sit-ups, and then finish up with, (6) light stretching for 3 minutes.

As your fitness level improves, the daily endurance and flexibility activities will continue, and you will be adding different strength exercises as well as your favorite physical activities in order to develop coordination and keep the program a varied and interesting one.

Name: _____   Beginning Weeks   Date: _____

	MON	Key Min	TUES	Key Min	WED	Key Min	THUR	Key Min	FRI	Key Min	SAT	Key Min	SUN	Key Min
1	Jog-Walk-Jog	E 3	Jog	E 3	Jog-Walk-	E 3	Jog	E 3	Jog-Walk-Jog	E 3	Cycling	E 30	Walk	R 3
2	Stretch	F 10	Stretch	F 10	Stretch	F 10	Stretch	F 10	Stretch	F 10	Stretch	F 5	Stretch	F 5
3	Jog	E 10	Jog-Walk-Jog	E 12	Jog	E 10	Jog-Walk-Jog	E 12	Jog	E 10	Sit-ups (10x)	S 12	Walk	E 25
4	Stretch	F 5	Stretch	R 5	Stretch	R 5	Sit-ups (10x)	S 3	Stretch	F 5				
5			Sit-ups (10x)	S 2	Coordination (8-count arm)	C 3	Stretch	F 5	Calisthenics (8-count arm)	C 2				
6			Stretch	E 3										
Total Time	28		35		31		33		30		47		33	

Key:
E = Endurance   (walking/jog-walk-jog/walk-jog-run/running/intervals/swimming)
                  (cycling/rowing/cross-country skiing/climbing/aerobic dance/rope skip)
F = Flexibility   (stretching/yoga/passive manipulation/calisthenics)
S = Strength   (calisthenics/weight training/gymnastics/universal gym/circuit training)
C = Coordination (calisthenics/trampoline/volleyball/racquetball/handball/tennis/table tennis)
R = Relaxation   (progressive relaxation exercises/sauna/whirlpool/jacuzzi/steamroom/swimming)

Name: Date:

Three-Month Level

	MON	Key/Min	TUES	Key/Min	WED	Key/Min	THUR	Key/Min	FRI	Key/Min	SAT	Key/Min	SUN	Key/Min
1	Jogging	E 5	Jog-Walk-Jog	E 5	Jogging	E 5	Jog-Walk-Jog	E 5	Jog	E 5	Jog-Walk-Jog	E 5	Stretch	F 3
2	Stretch	F 10	Stretch	F 10	Stretch	F 10	Stretch	F 10	Stretch	F 10	Stretch	F 5	Cycling	E 35
3	Jogging	E 15	Jogging	E 2	Jog	E 18	Jog or Swim	E 12	Walk-Jog-Run-Jog	E 20	Volleyball/Tennis/Racquetball (choice)	C 25	Sit-ups (20x)	S 5
4	Sit-ups (15x)	S 5	Push-ups	S 5	Sit-ups (20x)	S 10	Push-ups (10x)	S 5	Sit-ups (20x)	S 3	Pull-ups (3x)	S 5		
5	Stretch	F 5	Stretch	F 5	Stretch	F 5	Stretch	F 5	Stretch	F 5	Stretch	F 5		
6	8-count arm-ex	C 3		R 10	8-count arm ex	C 2			8-count arm ex	C 3				
Total Time	43		32		45		35		48		42		43	

Key: Same as Beginning Weeks.

Name: Date:

Six-month level

	MON	Key Min	TUES	Key Min	WED	Key Min	THUR	Key Min	FRI	Key Min	SAT	Key Min	SUN	Key Min
1	Jog	E 5	Jog	E 5	Jog	E 5	Jog	E 5	Jog	E 5	Jog	E 5	Stretch	F 3
2	Stretch	F 10	Stretch	F 10	Stretch	F 10	Stretch	F 10	Stretch	F 10	Stretch	F 10	Sit-ups (25x)	S 7
3	Sit-ups (20x)	S 5	Sit-ups (20x) Push-ups (15x)	S 5 / 5	Pull-ups (5x)	S 5 / 5	Sit-ups (20x) Push-ups (15x)	S 5 / 5	Sit-ups (20x) Push-ups (15x)	S 5 / 5	Pull-ups	S 5	Walk or Cycle	E 55
4	Jog	E 20	Tennis	C 25	Run 10 x 300 @ 75 sec w 100 m walk	C 25	6-count foot	C 1	Volleyball	C 25	Run 5–6 mile or Compete	E 40		
5	8-count arm 6-count foot	C 2 / 2	Jog	E 10	Stretch (achilles)	E 10	Run	E 35	Jog	E 5	Rope-skip	C 3		
6			Stretch	F 3		F 3	Stretch (achilles)	F 3	Stretch	F 3				
Total Time	**44**		**63**		**51**		**64**		**58**		**63**		**65**	

Key: Same as beginning level.

Name: Nine-month level   Date:

	MON	Key Min	TUES	Key Min	WED	Key Min	THUR	Key Min	FRI	Key Min	SAT	Key Min	SUN	Key Min
1	Jog	E 5	Jog	E 5	Jog	E 5	Jog	E 5	Jog	E 5	Jog	E 5	Stretch	E 5
2	Stretch	F 10	Stretch	F 10	Stretch	F 10	Stretch	F 10	Stretch	F 10	Stretch	F 10	Sit-ups (30x)	S 10
3	Sit-ups (30x) Push-ups (20x)	S 8	Sit-ups (30x) Push-ups (20x)	S 8	Sit-ups (35x) Pull-ups (7x)	S 8 / 5	Sit-ups (35x) Pull-ups (7x)	S 8 / 5	Sit-ups (35x) Push-ups (25x)	S 8 / 5	Sit-ups (40x)	S 3	Run or Cycle	E 45 / 50
4	Walk Jog-Run	E 30	Tennis or Handball	E 30	Volleyball	C 30	Tennis or Racquetball	C 15	Run 8 x 440 s @ 95 w 220 w	C 35 / 30	Tennis Racquetball or Handball	C 40 / 30 / 30		
5	Rope Skip	C 2	Jog-Walk-Jog	C 2	Run	E 10	Jog-Walk-Jog	E 30	Ropeskip	C 2	Run	C 10		
6									Stretch	R 10	Stretch	F 3		
Total Time		60		73		73		60		50		61		65

Key: Same as beginning level.

Name: Twelve-month level   Date:

	MON	Key / Min	TUES	Key / Min	WED	Key / Min	THUR	Key / Min	FRI	Key / Min	SAT	Key / Min	SUN	Key / Min
1	Jog	E 5	Jog	E 5	Jog	E 5	Jog	E 5	Jog	E 5	Jog	E 5	Push-ups (20x)	S 7
2	Stretch	F 10	Stretch	F 10	Stretch	F 10	Stretch	F 10	Stretch	F 10	Stretch	F 3	Stretch	F 3
3	Sit-ups (35x)	S 10	Sit-ups (35x) Pull-ups (10x)	S 10 / 5	Sit-ups (40x)	S 10	Sit-ups (40x) Pull-ups (10x)	S 10 / 5	Sit-ups (50x)	S 15	Sit-ups (25x)	S 7	Tennis Racquetball or Handball	C 30
4	Run	E 30	Run	E 30	Run or Swim	E 35 / 15	Run 12 x 220 @ 45 w 220 walk	E 20	Run	E 30	Run or Compete	E 45	Jogging or Cycling	E 10 / 30
5	Stretch	F 5	Stretch (achilles)	F 3			Stretch	F 3						
Total Times		60		63		50		53		60		60		60

Key: Same as beginning level.

8
Injuries and Precautions

"An ounce of prevention is not enough," and "a pound of cure probably won't restore." These turns of old adages approach the essential requirements for keeping muscles, tendons, and joints healthy. This chapter will deal with problem areas where injury is common—yet avoidable, with understanding, motivation, and patience.

Regardless of the type of activity in which you choose to engage, you will always depend a great deal on your legs to hold you up and to get you there. Thus, physically active people have more problems with legs than with all other areas put together.

Foot and Ankle

When a person has not exercised regularly for a period of months or years, the joints of the lower extremities are very vulnerable to the stress of daily vigorous physical activity.

Sprain

Sprains are the most common injuries of physical activity. They are caused by a sudden overstretching of tendons or ligaments, resulting in the fibers tearing: bleeding, pain, and swelling develop. The degree of these symptoms indicates the severity of the sprain, and the amount of discomfort later tells us whether it is serious enough to curtail or discontinue regular training.

Although rough, uneven surfaces strengthen the muscles and toughen tendons and ligaments, they also cause sprains and therefore should be avoided until full recovery occurs, or in general until the muscle-tendon-ligament complex has been sufficiently strengthened by the training program. Slow and patient progression to former training levels will allow the structures of the foot and ankle to recover. Proper footwear, accompanied by sufficient warm-up, is another important feature in the prevention and correction of sprains. Ice, elevation, and compression are the standard treatments for sprains and should follow the injury as soon as possible.

Stress Fractures (March Fractures)

These can occur in the foot or leg subjected to repeated pounding without adequate protection, and from gradual or rapid increase in training loads. Stress fractures are hairline breaks in the bones caused by the accumulative effects of micro-movements within the bone as a result of thousands of jarrings. It is similar to the effect of bending a small piece of wire many times until it breaks. Often these fractures are so small that they are not identified in x-rays until weeks after they occur. They show up well in the x-ray picture later when calcium deposits of the new bone cells are laid down. Rest and/or casting is usually prescribed to allow complete recovery.

Tendonitis

Tendonitis (an inflammation of the sheath that surrounds the tendon as it passes over a joint or through a narrow passage) is a common difficulty among dedicated athletes. Training too hard too soon is usually the cause of this ailment as with other running injuries. This, too, can be avoided by slow, gentle progression toward heavier training loads. One feels tenderness and pain with pressure or movement. It occurs most frequently in the Achilles tendon just above the heel; on top of the foot arch where the extensor tendons pass on their way to the toes; and on both sides of the ankle joint where tendons pass.

Tendonitis is one of the most difficult injuries to cure. The athlete has the choice of easing up and diminishing the intensity and duration of his exercises, or stopping training altogether. Neither choice is guaranteed to eliminate the problem. The symptoms of tendonitis arise from friction: a rubbing of the inflammed tendon as it slides through its covering sheath. Eventually, the body warns us that it is "too much too soon and something has got to change." Often slight changes in rou-

tine for a few days can give the offended area a chance to
recover. If the tendonitis is accompanied by a swelling, tenderness, or crepitation (grating sound or feeling), cessation of
training and medical attention are needed. Sometimes a cast is
necessary for several days to rest the injured areas completely.

Blisters

Blisters are sometimes regarded as a "badge of courage" by
the weekend athlete. However, if you wish to make physical
activity an integral part of your everyday life, then blisters are
to be avoided, and once they occur they should be treated
seriously. Blisters, which are caused by friction between the
skin and shoes, can result in related injuries at joints far from
the scene of the blister. The discomfort of a blister on the foot
can throw off stride and posture, and thus exert unnatural
pressure and strain on the knee, hip, or back. Well-fitting shoes,
thin seamless socks, and trimmed toenails are good preventive
measures. Other precautions are: (1) applying a lubricant
around the toes and all areas that rub against other surfaces,
(2) painting the tender areas with tincture of benzoin, which
helps toughen the skin, and then using powder on the toes,
(3) wrapping the most vulnerable areas with thin elastic gauze
under a couple of layers of tape. Of course, our standard admo-
nition is appropriate here, too: *Start training slowly and build
up gradually.*

Shin

The term "shin splints" has been used to describe anything
that hurts between the knee and the ankle on the front of the
unbroken leg. The pain and disability of shin splints can be mild
or so severe as to be completely disabling. The causes of this
symptom are varied and obscure: overuse of the anterior
muscles, weak or unstable feet, improper shoes or hard surfaces,
and sometimes muscle imbalance between the strong flexor (in
the back of the lower leg) and weaker extensors (in the front
of the lower leg). Sometimes the malady occurs unannounced
and the victim is unable to identify the cause. Usually increasing the intensity or duration of the physical activity or training

on a new kind of surface is the culprit. Shin splints can occur in the well-conditioned athlete as well as in unconditioned individuals.

The two most common sites of this injury are: (1) the medial (inside) ridge of the tibia about midway between the knee and the ankle, and (2) the lateral (outside) side of the tibia, a bit above where the muscle that lifts the foot upwards attaches to the bone. The condition may be caused by small muscle or tendon tears which pull away from the bone; the consequent swelling causes the pain and limitation of motion.

Prevention of shin splints is based on a slow, progressive warm-up, including a great deal of stretching of the foot and ankle in every direction. Begin with a couple of laps of slow jogging, then sit on the ground with legs spread and extended (A). Support the trunk with the hands resting on the ground behind the back, then begin slowly to move the feet in gradually increasing circles with the heels remaining on the ground. It is important to keep pushing the joints as far as they will go to maintain maximum range of motion in all directions.

After several minutes of this ankle manipulation, pull the feet up behind you with hands on knees, and sit on your heels with toes pointed to the rear. Stay in this position for a few minutes to allow the muscles to relax and the tendons to stretch. Now stand up and lean on a fence or post. Place one foot behind you as far as you can, keeping the heel on the ground. Now, while leaning forward, push backward on the rear foot, keeping the back knee straight, thus stretching the structures in back of the ankle and lower leg. Exaggerated pigeon-toed walking may also be effective to relieve shin splints.[49]

Whenever you make a change in your exercise routine, such as increasing the intensity, duration, or type of surface you are used to, make certain that your changes are minimal and gradual. When changing from a wooden floor to concrete, or from grass to asphalt surface, take it easy for a few days until the structures of the leg have a chance to adapt to the new conditions. If given half a chance, the body can adapt to virtually any kind of stress or change.

The immediate treatments of shin splints are ice, elevation, and rest. Thereafter, you can do several things that reduce the stress on the sensitive structures. Placing felt pads under the heel may take the strain off the tendon (tibialis posterior) located on the inner side of the shin and ankle. A couple of pieces of tape pulled up firmly around the instep may prevent irritation to the muscle (tibialis anterior) originating on the upper third of the lateral aspect of the tibia and crossing the top of the ankle. Another treatment is to wrap the lower third of the leg with thin sponge and tape it in place. Because the lower portion of the leg is made up primarily of bone, tendon, and fascia, its blood supply is minimal. The swelling that takes place within the walls of an irritated tendon sheath can restrict the circulation even further and cause prolonged disability.

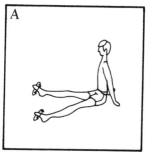

Knee

Knee injuries or symptoms are frequently caused by problems originating elsewhere: differences in leg length, foot disorders, improper shoes, uneven running surfaces, and leg muscle imbalance. Repeated incorrect foot placement, especially during prolonged activity, can transmit injury producing forces to the knee, which is the body's most insecure joint.

The vulnerability of the knee results from its anatomical complexity and its limited blood supply. Most of the nourishment to the knee comes from the synovial fluid that bathes the joint. Frequent straining of small ligaments attaching the semilunar cartilages (small quarter-moon shaped structures that cradle the lower end of the femur on top of the tibia) to the top of the tibia causes discomfort during weight-bearing activity. Tendonitis of the major tendon crossing the front of the knee over the kneecap can be caused by extended exercise periods, poor body mechanics, or direct injury caused by bumping, twisting, or stepping in a hole unexpectedly.

Once a knee is injured enough to restrict movement, the thigh muscles begin to atrophy (shrink) almost immediately. This starts a vicious cycle because the weakened muscles result in additional strains on the knee joint. One way of breaking the cycle (or preventing it) is to strengthen the quadriceps muscle (the large muscle group on the front of the thigh) with specific knee extension exercises. Repetitions of knee extensor exercises with weights on the feet can help to restore the muscles to previous or even greater strength (B). Another effective means of "training through" a knee injury is to run uphill fairly hard, and avoid slow jogging or downhill running. Effective treatment methods include: individually fitted foot supports; proper running shoes (firm heel counter and ½-inch heel, solid shank, and triple-layered soles); lifts for a leg of unequal length; flexibility exercises for the calf, hamstrings and Achilles tendons; and ice packs.

Hip

Injuries to the hip are relatively uncommon. The anatomical structure of the hip joint is very strong, and is supported by many large muscles. Hip injuries are usually short-lived and amenable to treatment.

Long distance runners and cyclists often suffer from bursitis of the hip, especially following a period of over-training. Rest, and sometimes medication, usually corrects the problem without difficulty. Incorrect posture, though it has the potential to cause hip problems, is more often transmitted to the knee joint. Exercises that stretch the hip and groin area before strenuous exercise will prevent most hip injuries. Easy jogging on soft surfaces can help heal an injured hip by increasing its blood supply.

Trunk

Low back trouble can be caused by poor body mechanics or from a poor balance between certain muscle groups. If one leg is shorter than the other (hereditary, or due to faulty or worn footwear), it will transmit stresses through the spinal column. Sudden twisting movements may cause excessive pressure on the spinal discs or cause minute tears in muscle tissue. These will be experienced as muscle spasms with considerable pain. The most common cause of low back pain in physically active people is weakness of abdominal muscles, worsened by tightness of the hip flexor and low back muscles.

If you are susceptible to low back pain you must pay special attention to the proper mechanics of walking, running, lifting, and sleeping, but first you must do what you can to minimize the risks. First, emphasize stretching exercises for the lower back and the front of the hips. For example, an excellent extensor exercise is the following: lay on your back and bend and grasp the knees with your hands. Then pull your knees toward the shoulders, slowly but firmly to the limit (C). Then raise your head toward the knees and hold this position for the count of ten. Finally, let your legs down slowly until your feet are flat on the ground. Repeat this ten times and do it three times each day.

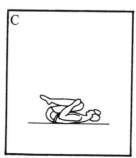

An exercise for the hip flexors that increases their range of motion is accomplished with stretching of the Achilles tendon as described previously. Another effective hip exercise, one which stretches the anterior thigh muscles, is to sit on the heels and gradually incline the torso backward until it is parallel with the lower legs. Stretching exercises for the inside of the groin are described in Chapter 7. Most low back problems can be helped by doing "bent-knee" sit-ups and the pelvic tuck exercise.

Abdominal injuries or pain can be divided into two categories: those involving the abdominal wall muscles, and those involving internal organs. The slight abdominal muscle tears that occur during vigorous activity usually do not prevent continued participation.

Muscle cramps that commonly afflict athletes can be avoided by proper warm-up, including stretching. When a muscle spasm does occur, the simplest and most effective solution is to place the spastic area on maximal stretch. If it is the abdominal muscles, hang from an overhead bar or reach as high as possible five or ten times (sometimes leaning to the side with arms outstretched). If the spastic area is toward one side of the trunk, then bend slowly in the opposite direction to place these muscles on maximum stretch.

Nonspecific pains within the abdominal cavity are of varied and often unknown cause. Indigestion accompanied by gas frequently inhibit the athlete from performing up to his potential. Avoiding air swallowing and gas-producing foods are useful preventive measures. Helpful solutions to the symptom are to bend toward the area of pain, flex the thighs to the chest, or massage the overlying muscles with the fingers.

The respiratory complex includes the rib cage, diaphragm muscles, and other muscles of the back and upper extremities. Relief from discomfort related to the mechanics of respiration may be obtained by conscious breath control. The common "stitch" in the side is probably caused by a spasm of the diaphragm muscle. If the circulatory system has not been opened up by proper warm-up activities, then adequate oxygen supply and waste removal in these muscles does not occur. Increasing the duration and intensity of the expiratory phase (exhalation) of breathing can help solve the "stitch" problem in two ways; it allows the diaphragm muscle a longer rest period and provides for a more complete removal of waste products.

The intercostal muscles that raise and lower the ribs can also suffer minor strains during vigorous physical activity. A common area is under or below the shoulder blades. Recovery is usually rapid, if a shift is made to light training for a few days, because heavy breathing aggravates the problem.

Part Three:
Dieting:
The Do's and Don'ts

9
Nutrition
and Health

Nutritional Requirements

Humans require various amounts of approximately 50 different nutrients within the major classes of foods: proteins, carbohydrates, fats, minerals, and vitamins. Precise amounts cannot be determined because humans, as well as animals, differ individually in their need for these nutrients. The range of differences (biological individuality) may be as great as 300%.[50] Also, tests for adequacy have been based to a considerate extent on acute and obvious deficiencies rather than optimal levels of nutrients. No reliable test for determining human requirements has yet been devised. Furthermore, most research has been with animals, and we do not know for certain the degree of applicability to humans.

Despite these limitations two standards have been developed: Minimum Daily Requirement (MDR) and Recommended Dietary Allowance (RDA). The MDR's were established by the Food and Drug Administration and are average levels required to prevent symptoms of actual deficiency with a small safety margin. The RDA's were developed by the Food and Nutrition Board of the National Academy of Sciences and are higher than the MDR's, allowing for: variation among individuals, the lack of precision of the tests of adequacy, and the assumption that "amounts above minimal confer added benefits to health."[51]

Our optimal diets fulfill the RDA's for all nutrients. Therefore, knowing specific RDA's is not necessary for using the Optimal Diet.

Variety

A major principle of nutrition is variety. Variety helps to ensure that the individual has an ample supply of all 50 nutrients. Fortunately, most nutrients are rather widespread through foods, so we have been able to function well on a wide variety of diets.

One of the most common errors made in eating habits, and a major cause of deficiencies, is preference for a few foods and a near exclusion of other foods. Many deliberately limit their selection to the foods they assume are "low calorie." Actually, it is unsafe to be so restrictive, and an effective and safe reducing diet requires variety.

Taste, Appearance

Americans have become accustomed to selecting foods that have had salt, sugar, or fat added to "improve" taste. Expenditures for snack foods have increased by 60% and soft drinks by 80% over the past 20 years.[52]

● Most canned vegetables have had salt added, and many of them sugar.

● The snack foods have both sugar and fat. The innocent looking potato chip contains most of its calories as fat.

● A major ingredient of Granola is vegetable oil, which is fat high in calories.

● A favorite pastime is a trip to a "fast-food" restaurant for french fried taste treats.

● Bacon and eggs have become synonymous with breakfast.

Although these foods are largely left out of the Optimal Diet, we need not fear being subjected to tasteless, uninteresting food. There are many recipes that meet the requirements of the Optimal Diet: Appendix B lists a few of these. In fact, conversion to the Optimal Diet opens a new world of taste. We have found that in time most people begin to prefer nonfat milk, unsalted vegetables, cereal without sugar, and foods cooked without fats. Our tastes can change. Have you tried steamed vegetables, or vegetables hot out of the pressure cooker? Do you know the delicious flavor and smell of homemade bread, hot out of the oven? Have you tried baked fish recipes using lemon juice, wines, and various condiments? Have you looked at gourmet recipes using fowl and various rice recipes?

Food can lose taste and appearance if improperly handled. Appendix D offers some tips to preserve and enhance taste.

When you convert to the Optimal Diet, you have to notice what you eat, and you will find that a new awareness will open to you.

Food Preservation

Food can lose taste, appearance, and nutritional value if improperly preserved. Yet food preservation is not a complicated art. Appendix C, "Food Preservation Tips," offers some ideas to preserve food and enhance its taste. You will find that attaching these sheets to your refrigerator will help you master the techniques.

The Optimal Diet should not increase your food bill. Because pastries and other unhealthy snacks are relatively expensive, your costs will actually decrease. A U.S. Department of Agriculture study showed that many "poor" families were eating an excellent diet. However, there are numerous other ways to save money while eating optimally well. Some of these ways are listed later in this chapter: Shopping for Optimal Nutrition.

Snacking; Sugar

Snacking is one of our favorite pastimes and strongest habits— the coffee and pastry breaks in the morning, perhaps beer and pretzels in the evening. These snacks are empty food, low in nourishment. But this does not mean we must give up all snacking. Chapter 10 and Appendix C contain many snacks that provide excellent nourishment.

To make effective use of these lists, it is well to make a point of including some of their contents in your weekly grocery purchase so that they are available when you get the urge to snack. Note that these snacks are all low in calories.

American sugar consumption averages about 500 calories per day, or up to 120 pounds per year. These are "empty calories," i.e., devoid of minerals, vitamins, and proteins. This means that almost all of our essential nutrients must be obtained from the remainder of our diet. Therefore, malnourishment is one of the potential problems of excessive sugar intake. Furthermore, excessive sugar in the diet has been implicated in some studies as a factor in heart disease.[53] In these studies the average sugar intake of 22 countries was compared. A high correlation

between levels of dietary sugar and incidence of heart disease
was found. High sugar intake has also been found to increase
blood cholesterol and triglycerides in some people.[54]

Avoiding these problems poses a special problem for Americans because of the prevalence of sugar in many processed foods
—soups, canned vegetables, and salad dressings—which is aggra-
vated by its availability, taste appeal, and mass-media advertis-
ing. Many people find it easier to abstain from sweets by
substituting a variety of tasty snacks, free of sugar.

Food Processing

The "health foods" industry has expressed concern about
dangerous food additives and the removal of essential nutrients
during the processing of foods. It raises the spectre of pesti-
cides, foreign chemicals in foods, the denuding of food in the
milling and canning processes, and destruction of the vital
properties of food.

There are 50 known nutrients in foods, and most of them are
very stable. Three classes of food, *proteins, carbohydrates,* and
fats, will be changed very little whether you freeze, eat raw,
cook, can, or smoke them. The amino acids of proteins remain
unchanged unless you burn them to cinders. Cooking meats
and starch foods improves their digestibility slightly.

The fourth food class, *minerals,* is even more stable, though
up to 20% may be dissolved by cooking water if improperly
cooked. Some *vitamins,* the fifth class of foods, have some
instability, but the freezing and canning process is more likely
to preserve these vitamins, than other food-handling techniques.
Certain vitamins have instabilities to light, air, and heat. The
food processing industry and government agencies that oversee
them are well aware of these instabilities and take great care to
preserve nutrients in food processing techniques.

Food additives. Food additives are for preservation and taste.
These chemicals are frequently found naturally in foods or
naturally in the human body. In any case, these substances must
be tested on various animals at levels 150 or more times as high
as humans would eat, without harmful effect, before they are
approved by the Food and Drug Administration.

There has been much publicity of late on the dangers of food additives. Health food alarmists refer to them as chemical poisons. Some of this concern was accentuated during the cyclamate controversy. Cyclamate was eventually banned by the Pure Foods and Drugs Administration (FDA) based on experimental studies in which it produced cancer in some mice. What may not be generally understood was that mice were fed amounts of cyclamate 150 times in excess of even the most avid eaters of cyclamate. In the opinion of some nutritionists, cyclamate should not have been banned.

There is also danger in excessive amounts of "natural foods." Too much carrot juice high in vitamin A can kill you. The level of iron that begins to be toxic for men is about five times our average daily intake. Alcohol can kill. Sugar can be a slow killer in excessive amounts by its effect on blood fat. Thus, continued concern and control over additives to natural foods whether they be synthetics (such as cyclamates) or natural foods themselves (sugar, salts, vitamins) is justified.

Supplements. Supplements of vitamins, minerals, and proteins are recommended almost exclusively by those who sell them. This is a billion dollar business based on uncertainty: "Could my diet be inadequate? Will vitamin C prevent colds? Perhaps vitamin E will extend my life. Maybe if I take a multiple vitamin each day, I won't have to worry." There is some danger in taking such supplements, i.e., accumulating too much of *certain* vitamins and minerals. The toxic amount of vitamin A, for example, is about 50,000 International Units per day, or 10 times the recommended dose for men. Selenium is essential to human life, but is more poisonous than arsenic. When we satisfy these needs from ordinary foods, we are protected from excess. But if we eat them in their pure states, as supplements, we may reach toxic amounts. Although moderate intake of vitamin or mineral supplements is not known to be dangerous, our optimal diets supply all nutrient requirements so that supplementary vitamins and minerals are not necessary.

Diet and Longevity

One hope of the human race is to find an answer to the prolongation of life. Generally speaking, whatever promotes our health and vigor will prolong our life. Therefore, a lifestyle that includes proper exercise, a nutritious diet in proper amounts, abstinence from cigarettes and drugs, avoidance of excessive stress, and a positive mental outlook, will promote health and long life. There have been many attempts to isolate specific nutrients, foods, herbs, or elixers that have special life-prolonging powers. Many claims have been made; none have been verified. We believe that good health and long life are a consequence of our overall lifestyle and genetic background.

10
The Optimal Diet

The typical U.S. diet is excessively high in cholesterol, animal fats (saturated), refined sugar (sucrose), salt, protein, and calories and too low in fiber and calcium. The emphasis on "adequate" amounts of eggs, meat, and dairy products—and on being a "good" (big) eater—is seen and felt everywhere. These eating habits are deeply ingrained in our culture among laymen, physicians, and nutritionists.

Diet, Atherosclerosis, and Heart Disease

During the past fifteen years, a vast and impressive amount of scientific evidence has accumulated implicating the American (U.S.) diet as a major factor in the causation of atherosclerosis. The link between diet, atherosclerosis, and coronary heart disease is based on the following evidence.[55]

- Severe atherosclerosis is the cause of most heart attacks (myocardial infarcts).
- The atherosclerotic plaque or lesion contains excessive amounts of cholesterol, which comes from the cholesterol in the blood.
- Sustained elevation of serum cholesterol from whatever cause is associated with a very high incidence of premature, severe atherosclerosis and coronary heart disease.
- The habitual ingestion of diets high in cholesterol and saturated fats is virtually a must for the development of significant atherosclerosis in a wide variety of experimental animals.
- The marked differences in serum cholesterol levels and coronary heart disease among different population groups are due to differences in dietary habits, as well as other living habits, rather than racial, ethnic, climatic, or geographic factors.

● In population groups with low mean serum cholesterol levels (125 to 175 mg%) the incidence of coronary heart disease and severe atherosclerosis is very low.

● High mean serum cholesterol levels (220 mg% or more) and high incidences of coronary heart disease (particularly in the middle aged) occur where diets are habitually high in cholesterol, total fats, saturated fats, and calories.

● Blood cholesterol levels can be significantly lowered by diets lower in cholesterol-saturated fats-calories.

The diet to replace the traditional one must satisfy the following criteria in order to merit the title of "Optimal" and be widely accepted:

● Contain much less cholesterol, animal fats, refined sugar, sodium, and calories.

● Be adequate in all food essentials.

● Supply sufficient variety of foods for life-long acceptability.

● Be attractive in taste and appearance.

● Contain readily available foods at a cost that does not exceed the diet it replaces.

The Optimal Diet vs. U.S. Diets

A comparison of the Optimal Diet (Table 10–1) with the usual U.S. diet reveals numerous differences. Note the markedly lower levels of total calories, fats (total and saturated), carbohydrates (total and refined), cholesterol, protein, and salt in the Optimal Diets. (Sample menus of the Optimal Diets are given at the end of the chapter.) Important differences from the usual U.S. diet are:

● Chicken, turkey, fish, and skim (nonfat) milk are the major protein sources, rather than eggs, beef, and veal, which are restricted to 1–3 times per week because of their higher content of saturated fat and/or cholesterol. Organ meats, pork, lamb, prime beef, luncheon meats, and shell fish, which are still higher in saturated fat and/or cholesterol are restricted still further (once per month).

● The same restriction is placed on concentrated sweets (candy, cakes, pies, etc.), ice cream, and other dairy products (except skim milk), and alcohol.

TABLE 10-1: NORMAL vs OPTIMAL DIET

		Normal	Optimal
Calories:	Total	3000 ± 500	1500 ± 500
	Meals	0–1500	250–600
	Snacks	50–600	50–150
Protein		100–160 gm	50–100 gm
Fat		120–140 gm (40–45%)	20–35 gm (15–20%)
Carbohydrate:	Total	250–350 gm (40–45%)	150–315 gm (60–65%)
	Sugar	15–30%	<15%
Cholesterol		600–1000 mg	<250 mg
Salt		10–20 gm	<5 gm
Calcium		<500 mg	800–1200 mg
Fiber		<10 gm	30–60 gm
Alcohol		Commonly used	Rarely used
Supplements		Commonly used	Rarely used

The Optimal Diet you choose depends on the calories required to achieve or maintain your optimal weight. This is a highly individual matter related to multiple factors, many of which are unknown. Thus, an estimate must be made (1000–2000 calories) based on the history of food intake, body weight as related to optimal weight, and physical activity. The final caloric level is arrived at by trial and error, based on the goal of achieving or maintaining optimal weight.

Our studies have shown that adult men and women who have achieved their optimal weight are able to maintain that weight on one of our optimal diets containing from 1000–2000 calories for periods of months to years.*

The amount of salt should be adjusted according to the presence or absence of hypertension and edematous states; e.g., patients with hypertension or edema should receive less than 2 gm of salt per day; those without these disorders may be given up to 5 gm of salt per day.

---

*It is interesting to note that in one of the author's recent studies, the inhabitants of Vilcambamba, Ecuador, who are famous for their longevity and freedom from heart disease, were found to consume an average diet of 1200 calories with 12–19% fat.[56]

The Optimal Diet is designed for all adults and children. Its caloric level must be adjusted from time to time depending on changes in the level of physical activity and the relationship of the actual weight to the optimal weight. The diet is specifically designed to prevent, control, or correct the common major metabolic disorders so prevalent in the U.S. Furthermore, all of our therapeutic diets are designed to simulate the optimal diet as closely as possible.

Optimal Diet Principles

The reader will note that the following diets differ markedly from the typical U.S. diet. They have substantially less total fat, saturated fat, cholesterol, protein, salt, meat, total and refined carbohydrate, and total calories. A much higher proportion of the fats is polyunsaturated (liquid vegetable oils—corn, cottonseed, safflower, sesame seed, soybean, and sunflower seed—which lower blood cholesterol). Other vegetable oils (olive, peanut) containing less polyunsaturated fat and not lowering serum cholesterol should be used sparingly; still others that are highly saturated (palm, coconut) should be avoided entirely.

Low-Cholesterol, Low-Calorie

The diets contain less than 300 milligrams of cholesterol—in contrast to the U.S. diet, which contains 600 to 1000 milligrams. The caloric level is considerably lower in the optimal diets (1000 to 2000) compared to the typical U.S. diet (2500 to 3500).

These differences from the usual U.S. diet are achieved by: 1) fewer eggs, less fat, no whole milk or dairy products made from cream or whole milk (ice cream, butter, whole milk cheeses); (2) smaller portions of poultry, fish, and meat (which is trimmed of all fat); (3) use of certain vegetable oils for cooking and salads; (4) avoidance of canned vegetables and soups, and preserved meats (bologna, salami, luncheon meats); (5) more fruits and vegetables.

Beverages

Because of the undesirable effects of caffeine on the heart, blood pressure, and blood sugar, we recommend restriction of coffee and tea to one cup or less per day. Instead, we suggest several coffee-like or noncaffeine coffee beverages. These beverages contain very little salt and calories, and are therefore suitable for all optimal and therapeutic diets. We also recommend drinking water with each meal or snack to help achieve an intake of at least 8–10 glasses (8 oz.) of fluids per day.

Vegetables

Over the past ten years our optimal diets have changed with respect to the amounts of animal products and plant foods: less and less meat and dairy products (especially those made from whole milk) to be replaced with more and more vegetables and fruits. At first this was done to decrease the amounts of saturated fat, cholesterol, salt, protein, and calories.

More recently there has been another reason for this trend in our thinking. The higher cost of animal foods in terms of production and land requirements in the face of the rapidly increasing world population will eventually make vegetarianism an economic necessity for all. Thus, we advocate the vegetarian diet several days per week.

Optimal Eating Habits

We have devoted much attention to *what* you should eat (the optimal diet). *How* you eat is also very important for optimal health. The following are our principles of optimal eating habits.

● Eat small, frequent meals rather than larger, fewer meals. We advocate feedings ranging from 250 to 600 calories for the three principle meals and 50 to 150 calories for the three between-meal snacks. The objective is to learn to eat just enough food to satisfy hunger rather than "filling up" to capacity.

● Strive to eat the minimal number of calories to obtain the essential nutrients you need to maintain your optimal body weight (primarily your optimal body fat) and vigor rather than the maximum number of calories you can eat without becoming overweight (excess fat).

● Try to eat in a certain place at a certain time and endeavor to do it in a quiet, friendly, relaxed atmosphere.

● Don't combine eating with other activities that result in a lack of awareness of what or how much you eat: TV-viewing, reading, or driving a car.

● Learn to eat slowly with many pauses and to savor each mouthful.

● Develop the habit of not adding salt or sugar to your foods and avoid foods to which these substances have already been added (packaged, preserved, or canned foods). Our optimal diets are made up of fresh foods and already contain sufficient salt and sugar for your nutritional needs. Excess (added) salt and sugar increase your risk for developing high blood pressure, heart disease, and stroke.

● Don't eat if you are very tired or emotionally upset. Delay your meal until you have at least partially recovered from these states.

OPTIMAL DIET 1 (1000 calorie plan)

Basic Menu Plan	Sample Menu A	Sample Menu B
BREAKFAST		
1 egg (2 per week only)	1 egg	1/2 cup oatmeal
1 fruit unit (list 2)	1/2 small grapefruit	1/2 cup orange juice
1 carbohydrate unit (list 3)	1 slice toast	1 slice toast
1/2 fat unit (list 5)	1/2 teaspoon margarine	1/2 teaspoon margarine
1/2 cup non-fat milk	1/2 cup non-fat milk	1/2 cup non-fat milk
water		
MID-MORNING		
water	hot tea with lemon	8 ounces diet lemonade
LUNCH		
1 ounce protein (list 4)	1 ounce baked chicken	1 ounce tuna
1 carbohydrate unit (list 3)	1 slice bread	1 slice bread
1/2 fat unit (list 5)	1/2 teaspoon margarine	1/2 teaspoon margarine
list 1 vegetables as desired	mixed green salad with tomato wedge/ vinegar dressing	1 cup cole slaw with green pepper rings
1 vegetable (list 3)	1/2 cup lima beans	1/4 cup baked beans
1 fruit unit (list 2)	1/2 cup fresh pineapple	1/2 cup cinammon applesauce
1/2 cup non-fat milk	1/2 cup non-fat milk	1/2 cup non-fat milk
water		
MID-AFTERNOON		
1 fruit unit (list 2)	small orange	2 fresh plums
water		
DINNER		
2 ounces protein (list 4)	2 ounces broiled halibut	2 ounces veal roast
1 carbohydrate unit (list 3)	1 slice bread	1 slice bread
1 list 3 vegetable	1 cup yellow squash	1 cup pickled beets
list 1 vegetables as desired	1 cup fresh broccoli	1 cup asparagus spears
1/2 cup non-fat milk	1/2 cup non-fat milk	1/2 cup non-fat milk
water	8 oz. coffee substitute	8 oz. coffee substitute
BEDTIME		
1 fruit unit (list 2)	1 large tangerine	1/2 cup sliced peaches

With Egg		Without Egg	
carbohydrate 54% calories	133 gm	carbohydrate 61% calories	148 gm
protein 22% calories	54 gm	protein 20% calories	49 gm
fat 23% calories	25 gm	fat 19% calories	20 gm
cholesterol	<450 mg	cholesterol	<200 mg
salt	<1.5 gm	salt	<1.5 gm

OPTIMAL DIET 2 (1200 calorie plan)

Basic Menu Plan	Sample Menu A	Sample Menu B
BREAKFAST		
1 egg (2 per week)	1 egg	1/2 cup oatmeal
1 fruit unit (list 2)	1/2 cup orange juice	1/2 cup applesauce
1 carbohydrate unit (list 3)	1 slice toast	1 slice toast
1/2 fat unit (list 5)	1/2 teaspoon margarine	1/2 teaspoon margarine
1 cup non-fat milk	1 cup non-fat milk	1 cup non-fat milk
water		
MID-MORNING		
water	6 ounces diet lemonade	iced tea with lemon
LUNCH		
2 ounces protein (list 4)	2 ounces ground beef	2 ounces tuna
1 carbohydrate unit (list 3)	1 slice bread	1 slice bread
list 1 vegetables as desired	1/2 teaspoon margarine	1/2 teaspoon margarine
1 list 3 vegetable	1 cup cole slaw with lemon juice dressing	tomato and cucumber salad with vinegar dressing
	1 cup green beans	1/3 cup lentils
	1/3 cup corn	
1 fruit unit (list 2)	1/2 cup fresh pineapple	1 large mandarin orange
1 cup non-fat milk	1 cup non-fat milk	1 cup non-fat milk
water		
MID-AFTERNOON		
1/2 carbohydrate unit (list 3)	2 melba toast	2 soda crackers
1 fruit unit (list 2)	1/2 cup apricots	1/2 cup sliced peaches
water		
DINNER		
2 ounces protein (list 4)	2 ounces baked fish	2 ounces roast turkey
1 carbohydrate unit (list 3)	1 small baked potato	1/2 cup steamed rice
list 1 vegetables as desired	1 cup fresh broccoli	1 cup brussels sprouts
	fresh tomato salad	large mixed green salad with tomato juice dressing
1 list 3 vegetable		
1/2 cup non-fat milk	1 cup carrots	1 cup turnips
water	1/2 cup non-fat milk	1/2 cup non-fat milk
BEDTIME		
1 fruit unit (list 2)	12 fresh grapes	1 small pear
beverage	coffee substitute	coffee substitute

	With Egg		Without Egg	
carbohydrate 54% calories	160 gm	carbohydrate 56% calories	175 gm
protein 24% calories	71 gm	protein 22% calories	66 gm
fat 22% calories	30 gm	fat 22% calories	30 gm
cholesterol	<450 mg	cholesterol	<250 mg
salt	<2 gm	salt	<2 gm

OPTIMAL DIET 3 (1500 calorie plan)

Basic Menu Plan	Sample Menu A	Sample Menu B
BREAKFAST		
1 egg (2 per week)	1 egg	1/2 cup cream of
1 fruit unit (list 2)	1/2 small grapefruit	wheat
2 carbohydrate units	1/2 cup oatmeal	1/4 medium canta-
(list 3)	1 slice toast	loupe
	1/2 teaspoon	2 slices toast
1/2 fat unit (list 5)	margarine	1/2 teaspoon
1 cup non-fat milk	1 cup non-fat milk	margarine
water		1 cup non-fat milk
MID-MORNING		
beverage	coffee substitute	coffee substitute
1 carbohydrate unit	4 unsalted crackers	1 slice toast
(list 3)		
LUNCH		
2 ounce protein (list 4)	2 ounce baked chicken	2 ounce ground beef
2 carbohydrate units	1/2 cup mashed potato	1/2 cup spaghetti
(list 3)	1 slice bread	1 slice bread
	1/2 teaspoon	1/2 teaspoon
1 fat unit (list 5)	margarine	margarine
1 vegetable unit	1 cup green peas	1 cup carrots
(list 3)	2/3 cup blueberries	1/2 cup fresh
1 fruit unit (list 2)	lettuce and tomato	pineapple
list 1 vegetables as	salad	large escarole and
desired		tomato salad/
1 cup non-fat milk	1 cup non-fat milk	vinegar dressing
water		1 cup non-fat milk
MID-AFTERNOON		
1 fruit unit (list 2)	1 small orange	2 medium plums
DINNER		
2 ounces protein	2 ounces lean beef	2 ounces broiled fish
(list 4)	roast	1 small baked potato
2 carbohydrate units	1/2 cup noodles	1 slice bread
(list 3)	1 slice bread	1/2 cup lima beans
1 vegetable unit	1/2 cup navy beans	cucumber and
(list 3)	fresh relish plate	endive salad
list 1 vegetables as	1 cup non-fat milk	1 cup non-fat milk
desired		
1 cup non-fat milk		
water		
BEDTIME		
1 carbohydrate unit	1 slice toast	4 melba toast
(list 3)	1/2 cup applesauce	1/2 cup orange juice
1 fruit unit (list 2)		

With Egg		Without Egg	
carbohydrate	211 gm	carbohydrate	226 gm
57% calories		60% calories	
protein	81 gm	protein	77 gm
22% calories		21% calories	
fat	35 gm	fat	30 gm
21% calories		18% calories	
cholesterol	<450 mg	cholesterol	<250 mg
salt	<2 gm	salt	<2 gm

OPTIMAL DIET 4 (1800 calorie plan)

Basic Menu Plan	Sample Menu A	Sample Menu B
BREAKFAST 1 fruit unit (list 2) 2 egg/week 2 carbohydrate units (list 3) 1/2 fat unit (list 5) 1 cup non-fat milk water	1/2 cup orange juice 1/2 cup cream of wheat 1 slice toast 1/2 teaspoon margarine 1 cup non-fat milk	1/2 cup grapefruit juice 1/2 cup oatmeal 1 slice toast 1/2 teaspoon margarine 1 cup non-fat milk
MID-MORNING 1 carbohydrate unit (list 3)	4 slices melba toast	1 slice toast
LUNCH 2 ounces protein (list 4) 3 carbohydrate units (list 3) 1 list 3 vegetable list 1 vegetables as desired 1 fruit unit (list 2) 1 cup non-fat milk water	2 ounces baked cod 1 small baked potato (4 oz.) 2 slices bread 1 cup green peas lettuce and tomato salad 1/2 cup pineapple 1 cup non-fat milk coffee substitute	2 ounces sliced chicken 1 1/2 cup steamed noodles 2 slices bread 1/2 cup navy beans fresh cucumber and tomato salad/ vinegar dressing 1 cup fresh water- melon cubes 1 cup non-fat milk coffee substitute
MID-AFTERNOON 1 carbohydrate unit (list 3) 1/2 fat unit (list 5) 1 cup non-fat milk water	4 soda crackers 1/2 teaspoon margarine 1 cup non-fat milk	1 slice toast 1/2 teaspoon margarine 1 cup non-fat milk
DINNER 2 ounces protein (list 4) 3 carbohydrate units (list 3) 1 list 3 vegetables list 1 vegetables as desired 1 cup non-fat milk 1 fruit unit (list 2) water	2 ounces roast turkey 1 cup mashed potato 1 slice bread 1/2 cup lima beans fresh relish plate 1 cup non-fat milk 1/2 cup orange sections	2 ounces lean roast beef 1 cup mashed potato 1 slice bread 1/2 cup pinto beans celery hearts/ radishes 1 cup non-fat milk 2/3 cup blueberries
BEDTIME 1 fruit unit 1 carbohydrate unit (list 3)	1 small pear 4 slices melba toast	1/2 cup orange juice 4 soda crackers

carbohydrate 63% calories	283 gm	fat 15% calories	30 gm	
protein 22% calories	97 gm	cholesterol (no egg)	<200 mg	
		salt	<2.5 gm	

OPTIMAL DIET 5 (2000 calorie plan)

Basic Menu Plan	Sample Menu A	Sample Menu B
BREAKFAST		
1 fruit unit (list 2)	1 cup orange juice	1 cup fresh apple-
2 1/2 carbohydrate	1 1/2 slice toast	sauce
units (list 3)	1/2 cup oatmeal	1 1/2 slice toast
2 eggs/week	1 teaspoon	1/2 cup cream of
1 fat unit (list 5)	margarine	wheat
1 cup non-fat milk	1 cup non-fat milk	1 teaspoon
		margarine
		1 cup non-fat milk
MID-MORNING		
1 cup non-fat milk	1 cup non-fat milk	1 cup non-fat milk
1 carbohydrate	4 pieces melba toast	1 slice toast
water		
LUNCH		
2 ounces protein	2 ounces sliced turkey	2 ounces tuna fish
(list 4)	1 cup steamed rice	2 slices bread
4 carbohydrate units	2 slices bread	1 cup beans
(list 3)	1/2 teaspoon	1/2 teaspoon
	margarine	margarine
1/2 fat units (list 2)	1 cup carrots	1 cup pickled beets
1 list 3 vegetable	cucumber and tomato	1 cup cucumbers/
list 1 vegetable as	salad with lemon	vinegar
desired	juice dressing	1/2 cup sliced
1 fruit unit (list 2)	1/2 cup pineapple	mangoes
water	chunks	coffee substitute
MID-AFTERNOON		
1 fruit unit (list 2)	1/2 cup applesauce	2/3 cup blueberries
water		
DINNER		
2 ounces protein	2 ounces ground beef	2 ounces baked
(list 4)	1 small baked potato	chicken
4 carbohydrate units	1 slice bread	1/2 cup mashed
(list 3)	2/3 cup corn	potato
	1/2 teaspoon	1 slice bread
1/2 fat unit (list 5)	margarine	2/3 cup lentils
1 list 3 vegetable	1 cup steamed	1/2 teaspoon
list 1 vegetable as	onions	margarine
desired	mixed green salad	1 cup green peas
beverage	coffee substitute	celery hearts and
1 cup non-fat milk	1 cup non-fat milk	radishes
water		1 cup non-fat milk
BEDTIME		
1 fruit unit (list 2)	1 large tangerine	1 small apple
1 cup non-fat milk	1 cup non-fat milk	1 cup non-fat milk

	carbohydrate	313 gm	fat	35 gm
	63% calories		16% calories	
	protein	101 gm	cholesterol	250 mg
	21% calories		(no egg)	
			salt	3.5 gm

Food Exchange List for All Diets

General Rules

1. Eat only foods listed on this diet, and in amounts indicated. Do not skip meals or feedings. Prepare and eat all food without added fat (oils, butter, margarine), sugar, salt, or gravy.
2. Use fresh or frozen meats, fish, fruit, and vegetables.
3. Salt and sugar substitutes may be used with your doctor's approval. Drink at least 1 glass of water before or with each meal.
4. Learn the caloric value of everything you eat.

List 1

Miscellaneous very low calorie foods: 25 calories per serving or less.

Seasoning: cinnamon, garlic, lemon, dry mustard, mint, nutmeg, parsley, pepper, sugarless sweeteners, spices, vanilla, vinegar, low-sodium tomato juice.

Salad Dressing: vinegar, lemon, pepper, parsley, garlic, salt substitute, dry mustard, and other spices.

Other foods: cranberries, diet soft drinks, decaffeinated coffee, coffee substitute (Postum, Breakfast Cup, Sanocaf, etc).

Vegetables: asparagus, broccoli, brussel sprouts, cabbage, cauliflower, cucumber, eggplant, lettuce, mushrooms, peppers, radishes, string beans, summer squash, tomatoes, watercress, wax beans, celery.

List 2

Fruit: 50 calories per serving.

apple	1 (2" dia.)
applesauce	1/2 cup
apricots	2 medium
banana	1 small
blueberries	2/3 cup
cantaloupe	1/4 (6" dia.)
cherries	10 large
grapefruit	1/2 small
grapefruit juice	1/2 cup
grapes	12
grape juice	1/4 cup
honeydew	1/8 (7")
mango	1/2 small
orange	1 small
orange juice	1/2 cup
peach	1 medium
pear	1 small

pineapple	1/2 cup
pineapple juice	1/3 cup
plums	2 medium
prune juice	1/4 cup
strawberries	1 cup
tangerine	1 large
watermelon	1 cup

List 3

Carbohydrate: 70 calories per serving

bread or tortilla	1 slice
roll	1 (2" dia.)
crackers	4 unsalted
cereals, cooked	1/2 cup
dry	3/4 cup
rice, grits, cooked	1/2 cup
beans, lima, navy	1/2 cup
baked	1/4 cup
spaghetti, noodles, macaroni	1/2 cup
corn, lentils, split peas	1/3 cup
potato, white	1 (2" dia.)
onions	1 cup
peas, green	1 cup
winter squash	1 cup
turnips, beets, rutabagas	1 cup
carrots	1 cup

List 4

Protein: 75 calories per serving

Eggs: Limit eggs to 2 or 3 per week. On other days substitute 1/2 cup cooked cereal or 3/4 cup dry cereal.

Meat: turkey, chicken, veal, lamb, beef: 1 slice (3" x 2" x 1/8" or 1 ounce).

Fish: bass, bluefish, catfish, cod, flounder, halibut, rockfish, salmon, sole, tuna (fresh, canned in water, or washed with water: same amount as meat). Fowl and fish are most desirable. Eat others only 1–2 times per week.

Low fat cottage cheese: 1/4 cup (use 1 portion only daily).

Non-fat milk, jello: 3/4 cup.

List 5

Fats: 45 calories per teaspoonful

Use 1 teaspoon special margarine (first ingredient liquid oil, corn, safflower, or soy), polyunsaturated cooking oil (corn or safflower), sauce or dressing made with corn or safflower oil.

Optimal Snacks

We are a nation of snack-eaters. At all hours of the day and night, at home, at work, at play, at all socioeconomic levels, we have the opportunity to eat, and have developed the habit of consuming many forms of foods and drinks in addition to the traditional three meal times.

This custom is so deeply entrenched in our way of life, it would be foolhardy to advise against it. Actually, the custom has advantages, and it is more logical and more fruitful to exploit these advantages than attempting to abolish the practice. Our objective is to establish optimal principles for making the best of an inevitable situation. The methods for doing this are:

1. To schedule the snacks at appropriate times of the day, individualizing them as necessary.

2. To improve the quality of the snacks by making them conform to the principles of our Optimal Diets. Indeed, we have employed these principles in designing our optimal and therapeutic diets; i.e., scheduling six food-intakes instead of the traditional three. The 6-feedings eating schedule has several advantages:

(a) Scheduled feedings are much more likely to conform to the principles of the Optimal Diet than unscheduled ones.

(b) In-between feedings serve to reduce excessive hunger at regular meal times, and thereby reduce the size of the regular meals.

(c) Frequent small meals help establish the habit of satisfaction with smaller amounts of food.

Choosing acceptable and available snacks poses problems because most of the popular ones are not acceptable; their content of cholesterol, saturated fats, sodium, refined carbohydrates, and calories is excessive. Nonetheless, there are a sizable number of acceptable snacks that can be readily carried along for in-between snacks. A list of commonly used snacks to be avoided or used only occasionally because they violate the principles of the Optimal Diet are given on page 125.

CALORIE RANGE: 50

Fruits and Juices

1 small apple *or* 1/2 cup fresh applesauce
2 fresh apricots *or* 4 dried unsweetened apricot halves
1/2 small banana
1 cup fresh strawberries *or* 2/3 cup fresh or frozen unsweetened blueberries
1/4 medium cantaloupe
10 large fresh cherries
1/2 small grapefruit
12 medium grapes
1 small orange
1 medium fresh peach *or* 1/2 cup canned unsweetened peach slices
1 small fresh pear *or* 1/2 cup canned unsweetened pear slices
1/2 cup fresh or canned unsweetened pineapple
2 medium fresh plums
1 large tangerine
1 cup cubed watermelon
1/2 cup fresh or canned unsweetened fruit cocktail
1/2 cup grapefruit juice
1/2 cup orange juice
1/3 cup apple juice
1/3 cup pineapple juice

Vegetables

1/2 cup mixed carrot and turnip strips
1/2 cup pickled beets with onion slices
1 cup sauerkraut with chopped green onion
4 cherry tomatoes with 1/2 cup carrot sticks
1/4 cup cooked carrots and 1/4 cup cucumber slices marinated in 2 teaspoons low calorie Italian dressing
1 cup marinated green beans with chopped green onions in 2 teaspoons low calorie French dressing
1/4 cup mixed kidney and green lima beans in 2 teaspoons low calorie Italian dressing

CALORIE RANGE: 50–100

Pear or peach half with 2 tablespoons cottage cheese (93)
2 dried prunes stuffed with 3 teaspoons unhydrogenated peanut butter (80)
1 ounce French or Italian bread sticks (92)
5 rye wafers (85)
5 ounce baked custard made with low cholesterol egg powder, artificial sweetener, and skim milk (78)
1/3 cup regular *or* 3/4 cup artifically sweetened gelatin dessert (70)

1/2 cup vanilla tapioca made with skim milk (70)

1 1/2 cups unbuttered popcorn (72)

1/2 cup dry unsugared cereal with 1/2 cup skim milk (87)

1/4 cup cottage cheese with 2 tablespoons artifically sweetened cranberry sauce (98)

1 cup hot beef consomme with 20 osyter crackers (70)

1 cup hot chicken broth with 3 bread sticks (70)

1 small corn muffin with 1 tablespoon artificially sweetened strawberry jam (80)

1 1/2 inch cube angle food cake with 1/2 cup fresh strawberries (90)

1 cup yoghurt made with skim milk (90)

1 cup skim milk buttermilk (88)

1 average size cooked chicken leg (90)

1/2 cup home baked beans with tomato sauce (100)

1 cup home-made popcorn with margarine (96)

1 medium size banana (100)

8 ounces gingerale (95)

CALORIE RANGE: 100–150

1 small French roll with 1 ounce chicken and chopped lettuce (115)

1 miniature corn taco (tacito) with 1 ounce shredded skim milk cheese and chopped lettuce (120)

large banana with 1/2 cup non-fat milk (133)

3 ounces cottage cheese with 1/2 cup mixed fresh fruit (149)

1 medium baked pear stuffed with 2 tablespoons raisins and 1/2 cup non-fat milk (133)

4 ounces baked pumpkin custard (150)

1 medium baked apple with 1/2 cup non-fat milk (137)

1/4 cup tuna salad with unsalted tuna, chopped celery, and 1 teaspoon safflower salad dressing (148)

1 6-inch matzo with 1 ounce skim milk cheese (140)

1 small hard roll with 1 ounce chopped turkey and chopped lettuce (135)

4 melba toast squares with 1 teaspoon special margarine (116)

2 tablespoons dry raisins with 2 graham crackers (108)

1 miniature hamburger with 1 small (1") roll and 1 ounce ground beef (120)

1 medium slice (3 x 4 x 1/4") cold roast beef (140)

Meritene Nog (120)—1/3 oz. Meritene Powder (plain, chocolate, or egg nog) mixed with 8 oz. non-fat milk

Shopping for Optimal Nutrition

1. Shop with an eye to getting the most nutritive value for your food dollar. Use the basic foods, meat, fish, poultry, dairy

products, fruits and vegetables, breads and cereals, but include non-fat milk and low-fat cottage cheese, more poultry and fish, more low salt, low calorie, polyunsaturated margarines and egg substitutes. Don't purchase fatty meats, pork products, highly saturated cheeses, whole milk, sugar, and cream.

2. Don't purchase foods that provide only "empty" calories, such as candy, snack foods, sodas, etc. Don't but these or any other food simply because you have a coupon or receive a premium. Unless the food meets good nutritional standards and provides some good nutrients, it is not a wise purchase.

3. Menus need not be expensive to be nutritious! But neither is an inexpensive meal a bargain if it is not eaten! Make sure the family begins early to enjoy a well-rounded meal that includes the basic foods. A meal filled with expensive "empty" foods may be woefully inadequate nutritionally.

4. Compare nutritive values, as well as price when you shop. A lean chuck roast may give you more nutritive value than a choice well-marbled steak, with fewer calories. A roasting chicken may end up being more nutritive and much less expensive than a prime rib roast with a 1 inch fat cover. Inexpensive less-tender cuts of meat are just as nutritive if braised or stewed. Only rarely purchase liver, kidney, sweetbreads, which have a high cholesterol level, and "luncheon" and delicatessen meats because their sodium and saturated fat levels are too high.

5. In many cases the best buy isn't always the cheapest! Compare quality as well as price. A pound of wilted string beans costing 15 cents that ends up being more string than bean, with no vitamin remaining after cooking, and left untouched on the family dinner plate, is not a bargain at any price.

6. Be sure to keep fresh food fresh after purchasing. The vitamin content of many foods may be diminished if food is not stored properly. When leftover cooked food is stored, be sure it is tightly wrapped to save nutrients. By the same token, cook fresh vegetables in small amounts of water, just until tender to avoid flavor loss, as well as loss of nutrients, and use the cooking water for sauces and soups.

7. Take a long hard look at convenience foods, particularly ready-to-use mixes. Serving for serving, these mixes are more

expensive than "from scratch" equivalents and may have some built-in hazards: The sodium level of most cake, cookie, pancake, and waffle mixes is high and the saturated fat level of items like pie crust and many frozen bakery products is equally so.

8. Be a label reader! Find out exactly what you are paying for. *Remember, the ingredient appearing first on a label of contents indicates that that particular item is present in the greatest quantity,* with all others in diminishing amounts. Learn to distinguish between saturated and unsaturated fats, vegetable oils, and hydrogenated products.

9. If a member of the family is on a special diet, compare the cost of packaged and canned "dietetic" food against fresh or frozen. Most specialty foods cost more and offer few advantages over fresh, except convenience. Also, bear in mind that calories can often be omitted simply by removing syrups from fruits, and by omitting sauces, gravy, and extra seasoning fats.

10. Use more herbs, dry and fresh, as well as lemon juice and flavored vinegars for dressings and seasonings, rather than the saturated salad dressings, whole-egg mayonnaise, and extra salt.

Selection Lists for Optimal Diets

MILK PRODUCTS

1 portion equals 1 cup or 8 ounces. Purchase fortified skim milk which has vitamins A and D added. Daily servings should include: 2–4 cups for children and teenagers, 1 1/2–3 cups for adults who are at or near optimal weight.

Recommended

Fortified skim or nonfat milk or fortified skim milk powder. Nonfat milks may vary in fat content from 0.1 to over 1%, and the label usually does not specify amount. We recommend nonfat milk powder, which contains the same amount of fat as nonfat milk, but is cheaper and can be made up in various amounts and dilutions to individual taste. Buttermilk made

Avoid or Use Rarely

Canned or whole milk, chocolate milk, ice cream, sour cream, half and half, sweet whipping cream, whole milk yoghurts. All nondairy cream substitutes that contain coconut oil high in saturated fat. All imitation milks that use coconut oil bases. All cheeses made from cream or whole milk. Butter.

from skim milk, yoghurt made from skim milk, evaporated canned skim milk, or cocoa made with low-fat milk. Imitation milk *only* if it contains corn, soybean, or safflower oils, and not a large concentration of coconut oil, as most of the present imitation milks now do.

Cheeses made from skim or partially skim milk, cottage cheese, preferably uncreamed, hoop cheese, farmer's or baker's cheese, Mozarella or Sap Sago cheeses.

EGGS AND EGG PRODUCTS

Recommended

Limit egg yolks to 2 or 3 per week; this is to include all eggs used in cooking. Count as part of daily and weekly allowance any cake, cookie, bread, batter, or sauce product that contains egg yolk. Egg whites do not contain fat, but have appreciable amounts of sodium. If sodium is restricted, then egg whites must be used sparingly.

MEAT, POULTRY, AND FISH, MEAT SUBSTITUTES

Recommended

Choose only lean cuts of meat and trim off all visible fat. Make selections from this list for the main (lunch or dinner) meals: *Poultry and fish* (skin removed): Choose from chicken, Rock Cornish hen, turkey, or squab; any type lean fish. From the meat substitutes choose uncreamed cottage cheese, partially skim milk, yoghurt, dried peas, beans, corn, or rice.

Make selections from the follow-

Avoid or Use Rarely

All fat, heavily marbled meats, fat short ribs, spare ribs, mutton, goose, duck, bacon, luncheon or delicatessen meats, all organ meats, liver, kidney, heart, sweetbreads (these are very high in cholesterol; however, because liver is very rich in iron and vitamins, a 4-ounce portion may be included in a meat meal once in a 2-week period). All shellfish including clams, crab, lobster, oysters, scallops, and shrimp are high in cholesterol, but low in

ing for only 1–2 meals/week (limit portions to 3 ounces):

Beef: lean ground chuck or ground round, sirloin tip, round, chuck, rump, or arm roast, or pot roasts, stew meat. Flank, sirloin, T-bone, or porterhouse, tenderloin, round or cube steaks. Shank or shin bone soup meat.

Lamb: leg meat for roast or steak, loin, rib or shoulder chops.

fat (a 4-ounce portion may be used as a substitute for meat once in a 2-week period).

Frankfurters, sausages, canned meats and fish packed in oil, bacon, salt pork, skin from turkey or chicken, all fish roes including caviar.

What Constitutes a Portion?

Each pound contains 16 ounces. For each 3-ounce portion of cooked meat, poultry, or fish allowed, count on purchasing an extra ounce or two to allow for shrinkage in cooking. Allow 2 ounces for meat with bone, 1 extra ounce for fish or lean meat without bone.

3-Ounce Portion Samples

A leg and thigh, or half breast of a 3 lb. chicken
2 (3 x 3 x 1/4 inch) slices roast beef
1 (3 x 1/2 inch thick) hamburger pattie

1-Ounce Portion Samples or Equivalents

1/4 cup chicken or turkey meat, loosely packed
1/4 cup tuna or salmon, water pack or washed of oil
4 tablespoons uncreamed cottage cheese
6 ounces plain yoghurt (3/4 container)
1/2 cup cooked dried beans or dried peas
8–10 walnuts (shelled)

VEGETABLES AND FRUIT

Recommended

Fresh, or frozen. Portion size 1/2 cup, with 3 or more portions allowed daily. At least 1 portion should be a source of vitamin C: broccoli, raw cabbage, berries, tomatoes, grapefruit or orange, cantaloupe, mango, melon, tangerine, papaya. At least 1 portion should be a source of vitamin A: broccoli, chard, carrots, chicory or escarole, beet, collard, dandelion, turnip or mustard greens, kale, peas, spinach, green beans, rutabaga, cress, winter squash, apricots.

Other fruits and vegetables are nutritious and should be eaten as salads, main dishes, snacks, and desserts, *in addition to* the recommended daily portions of the high vitamin A and C lists.

BREADS AND CEREALS

Recommended

Whole grain, enriched, or restored. One portion equals 1 slice; 1 portion of cereal equals 1/2 cup cooked or 3/4 cup cold or commercially prepared. This to include breads made with a minimum of saturated fat such as white enriched, whole wheat, raisin, English muffins, French and Italian breads, oatmeal, pumpernickel, rye, and homemade biscuits, muffins and griddle cakes made with liquid oil, hot and cold cereals, rice, melba toast, matzo, macaroni, noodles (except egg), and spaghetti.

Avoid or Use Rarely

Butter rolls, commercial biscuits, muffins, doughnuts, sweet rolls, or Danish rolls, cakes, crackers, egg bread, cheese breads, any commercial mix containing dried whole eggs or whole milk.

What Constitutes a Portion?

1 serving equals:
1 slice white, wheat, raisin, rye, brown, pumpernickel, French or Italian bread
1 3-inch roll
1 homemade biscuit or muffin (2–3 inches)
1 1-1/2 x 1-1/2 inch piece cornbread
1 4-inch griddle cake made with allowed oil and skim milk
4 pieces (3 x 1 1/2 x 1/8 inch) melba toast
1 (5 x 5 inch) matzo
3/4 ounce bread sticks or rye wafers
1-1/2 cups unsalted popcorn made with oil from day's allowance
1/2 cup cooked or 3/4 cup dry cereal
1/2 cup cooked rice, spaghetti, grits, barley, noodles, macaroni
1/4 cup dry bread crumbs
3 tablespoons white flour or 2-1/2 tablespoons dry corn meal
1 serving of these vegetable substitutes is equal to 1 portion:
1/2 cup cooked dried beans, peas, lentils, chickpeas, or garbanzos

1/3 cup whole kernel corn or cream style corn, or 1 4-inch ear of corn
1 small white potato or 1/4 cup cooked sweet potato
Note: Corn products, biscuits, waffles, griddle cakes and muffins contain more fat than other bread products. They may be used only if they are made at home with the allowed oil for the day, or as part of that allowance. Most crackers contain a significant amount of saturated fat, so are not recommended on the lower caloric levels.

FATS AND OILS

Recommended

All to be polyunsaturated. Depending on the caloric allowance, a range of 1–3 teaspoons per day in the form of margarine, oil, salad dressing or other polyunsaturated shortenings is allowed.

Use margarines, salad dressing and mayonnaise, liquid oil shortenings that contain any of these vegetable oils: corn, cottonseed, safflower, sesame seed, soybean, or sunflower seed.

Read the label on all products and choose those highest in polyunsaturates if one of the above oils appears *first* in the ingredients list, and one or more partially hydrogenated vegetable oils appears as an additional ingredient.

Avoid or Use Rarely

All solid fats and shortenings. Butter, lard, fat of salt pork and bacon, all solid fats from pork, beef, and lamb, completely hydrogenated margarines and vegetable shortenings, lard, all products containing coconut oil.

Peanut and olive oil may be used occasionally for flavor and variety, but *they do not take the place* of the recommended oils.

SUGARS, SWEETS, AND DESSERTS

Recommended

Acceptable for their low saturated fat and cholesterol level are: fresh fruit or canned unsweetened fruits, gelatin, water ices, fruit whips, puddings made with nonfat milk, sweets and bottled drinks made with cyclamate-free sweeteners, vinegar, dry mustard, herbs, and spices.

Avoid or Use Rarely

All coconut and coconut oil, commercial cake, pie, cookies, and mixes of each, frozen cream pies, eclairs and cream puffs, all commercially fried items such as fritos, potato chips and snack foods, whole milk puddings, chocolate pudding high in cocoa butter, all regular ice creams.

What Constitutes a Portion?

Each of the desserts below contain approximately 45 calories, and all are fat free:

1/4 cup prune or apricot whip

1/3 cup gelatin dessert

1/4 cup cornstarch or tapioca pudding made with fruit juice or with part of skim milk allowance

1/4 cup water ice

1/3 cup canned or frozen fruit (this is equal to 1 portion fruit and 1 tablespoon sugar)

1 small slice angel food cake

3 cornflake kisses or nut and cornflake meringues

Foods to Avoid

(Contain too much cholesterol, saturated fat, sodium, or refined sugar (display)

Animal fats

Avocados

Bacon, ham, pork

Bakery cakes of all kinds, or cake mixes (angel food excepted)

Butter crackers

Buttered, creamed or fried vegetables

Butter or products made with butter

Butter rolls, sweet rolls, cheese or egg rolls or bread

Canned meat products

Canned or dry soup

Cheese rolls or breads

Chocolate in any form

Coconut, coconut oil, palm oil, or olive oil

Commercial biscuits, biscuit mix

Commercial muffins, muffin mix, sweet roll mix, or frozen equivalents

Corned beef or pastrami

Corn, potato, or tortilla chips

Cream and sour cream blends or substitutes with coconut, palm, or a blend
  of both as a base (saturated fat)

Duck or goose

Fish roes, including caviar

French fried potatoes

French toast, pancakes or pancake mix, waffles or waffle mix

Frozen or packaged dinners

Granulated or powdered whole milk or powdered cream mixtures

Gravy, gravy mixes, cream sauces

Hydrogenated margarines
Luncheon meat, cold cuts, hot dogs, sausages, bologna, salami
Malted milk or blended malted milk powders
Nondairy creamers with coconut oil or palm oil
Olives
Organ meats, fresh or canned (liver, kidney, sweetbreads, brains)
Pies, including pie crust mixes
Peanut butter
Regular jams, jellies, and syrups, honey, and granulated sugars
Saturated shortenings and oils (hydrogenated)
Shellfish, fresh or canned
Spareribs
Sweetened, frozen, or canned beverages including carbonated drinks
Whipped cream, sour cream, 20- and 40-percent creams, coffee creams,
    half-and-half, regular ice cream, ice milk
Whole eggs or egg yolks
Whole milk cheeses, and cream cheese
Whole milk, condensed milk, evaporated whole milk
Whole milk yoghurt

11
Vegetarian Diet

History of Vegetarianism

Vegetarianism dates back thousands of years to several ancient oriental religions: Hinduism, Buddhism, Jainism, and Brahmanism. Historically, it has often resulted from necessity. The production of plant foods requires about half the land required for the production of animal foods. In the face of the threat of world hunger due to the population explosion, the time might come when necessity demands a return to the vegetarian diet by most of the world's people.

Many famous men have advocated vegetarianism: Pythagoras, Plato, Seneca, Plutarch, Milton, Newton, Pope, Voltaire, Rousseau, Shelley, Tolstoy, Ghandi, Shaw, Diogenes, Aristotle. A large majority of the world's population now subsists on predominantly vegetarian diets. In the U.S., vegetarianism began in 1817 with a branch of the Bible Christian Church in Philadelphia. Today, there are three distinct groups of vegetarians in the U.S.: some Roman Catholic orders (Trappists), the Seventh Day Adventist Church, and a miscellaneous group including adherents of Jainism and Zoroastrianism.

Vegetarian Diet Nutritional Value

There is an old nutritional belief that diets containing animal protein are necessarily superior to those composed of vegetable proteins. This concept was originally based on reports showing that physical and mental development and health of consumers of animal foods were generally superior to that of people on strictly vegetarian diets. Thinking now must be revised in light of more recent research on the nutritional value of plant proteins. Many studies have shown that several plant proteins can be used together so that the resulting mixture can have a higher nutritive value than the individual proteins alone. Supplementation of plant proteins with certain amino acids or the addition of milk and egg proteins (lacto and/or ovovegetarian diets) greatly improves the nutritional value of plant protein diets. Comparisons of meat protein and lacto-ovovegetarian diets have shown no clearcut difference in effects on metabolism, physiology, or endurance.[57] A number of studies have demonstrated the value of plant protein diets in the prevention and treatment of protein malnutrition in children.[58]

Vegetarian diets are lower in cholesterol and saturated fats, and associated with lower incidence of atherosclerosis and coronary heart disease.[59] From this standpoint, as well as that of decreasing world food supplies, the increased use of meatless diets is important to consider. Considerable research on the design of well-balanced, nutritionally complete, and tasteful plant food diets is in progress. We have found such diets useful for still another reason—weight reduction. They provide additional bulk in the low-calorie diet and thus are more filling and less stimulating to the appetite. We find that some obese individuals prefer them to conventional meat-containing low calorie diets.

Our diets are of the lacto-ovovegetarian type, and thus adequate protein content is readily achieved without amino acid supplementation. The large variety of vegetables and fruits makes possible a highly palatable diet for long-term use. We believe that alternation at various intervals of the vegetarian with the Optimal Diet is a good compromise for achieving optimal nutrition for many people. Our vegetarian diets are given at the end of this chapter at caloric levels of 560 to 2000.

VEGETARIAN DIET 1
(580 CALORIES)

Basic Diet Plan

Sample Menu

BREAKFAST
1 fruit (list 2)
1/2 carbohydrate (list 3)
1/2 cup non-fat milk
water

1/2 cup orange sections
1/2 slice toast
1/2 cup non-fat milk

MID-MORNING
1/2 cup non-fat milk

1/2 cup non-fat milk

LUNCH
1 egg or 1 ounce dairy protein
    (list 4)
1/2 carbohydrate (list 3)
list 1 vegetables as desired
1 fruit (list 2)
1/2 cup non-fat milk
water

1 scrambled egg
1/2 slice bread
1 cup cooked broccoli
large lettuce and tomato salad
1 small apple
1/2 cup non-fat milk

MID-AFTERNOON
1/2 cup non-fat milk

1/2 cup non-fat milk

DINNER
1 ounce dairy protein (list 4)
list 1 vegetables as desired

1 fruit (list 2)
1/2 cup non-fat milk
water

1 ounce cottage cheese
1 cup fresh asparagus
large cucumber and spinach salad/
    vinegar dressing
1/2 small banana
1/2 cup non-fat milk

BEDTIME
12 ounces diet drink

12 ounces diet lemonade

carbohydrate	76 gm	53% calories
protein	36 gm	25% calories
fat	14 gm	22% calories
cholesterol	<300 mg	
salt	<1.5 gm	

VEGETARIAN DIET 2
(1000 CALORIES)

Basic Diet Plan	Sample Menu

BREAKFAST

1 fruit (list 2)	1/2 small grapefruit
1 carbohydrate (list 3)	1 slice toast
1/2 cup non-fat milk	1/2 cup non-fat milk
hot beverage	coffee substitute
water	

MID-MORNING

1/2 cup non-fat milk	1/2 cup non-fat milk

LUNCH

1 ounce dairy protein or	1 poached egg
1 egg (list 4)	1 cup fresh broccoli
1/2 vegetable (list 3)	large mixed green salad/lemon
list 1 vegetables as desired	1/2 slice toast
1/2 carbohydrate (list 3)	1/2 teaspoon margarine
1/2 fat (list 5)	1/2 cup sliced peaches
1 fruit (list 2)	1/2 cup non-fat milk
1/2 cup non-fat milk	
water	

MID-AFTERNOON

1 fruit (list 2)	2 fresh plums

DINNER

2 ounces dairy protein (list 4)	2 ounces cottage cheese
1 carbohydrate (list 3)	1 small baked potato with
1/2 fat (list 5)	1/2 teaspoon margarine
1/2 vegetable (list 3)	1/2 cup steamed carrots
list 1 vegetables as desired	large tomato and endive salad
1 fruit (list 2)	1/2 cup fresh pineapple
1/2 cup non-fat milk	1/2 cup non-fat milk
water	

BEDTIME

1/2 cup non-fat milk	1/2 cup non-fat milk

carbohydrate	122 gm	51% calories
protein	50 gm	21% calories
fat	25 gm	22% calories
cholesterol	<450 mg	
salt	<2.5 gm	

VEGETARIAN DIET 3
(1200 CALORIES)

Basic Diet Plan	Sample Menu

BREAKFAST

1 fruit (list 2)	1/2 cup orange juice
1 carbohydrate (list 3)	1 slice toast
1/2 fat (list 5)	1/2 teaspoon margarine
1 cup non-fat milk	1 cup non-fat milk
beverage	coffee substitute
water	

MID-MORNING

1/2 cup non-fat milk	1/2 cup non-fat milk

LUNCH

2 ounces dairy protein (list 4)	2 ounces skim milk cheese
1 carbohydrate (list 3)	1 slice bread
1/2 fat (list 5)	1/2 teaspoon margarine
list 1 vegetable (list 3)	1 cup green peas
list 1 vegetables as desired	large cucumber and tomato salad
1 fruit (list 2)	1 small fresh pear
1 cup non-fat milk	1 cup non-fat milk
water	

MID-AFTERNOON

1 fruit (list 2)	1 small apple
water	iced or hot tea/lemon

DINNER

2 ounces dairy protein (list 4)	1 egg + 1 oz. skim milk cheese
1 1/2 carbohydrate (list 3)	1 small baked potato
1/2 fat (list 5)	1/2 slice bread
1 vegetable (list 3)	1/2 teaspoon margarine
list 1 vegetables as desired	1 cup carrots
1 fruit (list 2)	fresh relish plate
1 cup non-fat milk	1/2 small sliced banana
water	1 cup non-fat milk

BEDTIME

1/2 cup non-fat milk	1/2 cup non-fat milk

carbohydrate	174 gm	58% calories
protein	68 gm	23% calories
fat	25 gm	19% calories
cholesterol	<450 mg	
salt	<3 gm	

VEGETARIAN DIET 4
(1500 CALORIES)

Basic Diet Plan	**Sample Menu**
BREAKFAST	
1 fruit (list 2)	1/2 cup applesauce
1 carbohydrate (list 3)	1 slice toast
1/2 fat (list 3)	1/2 teaspoon margarine
1 cup non-fat milk	1 cup non-fat milk
water	
MID-MORNING	
1 fruit (list 2)	1/2 cup dried apricots
water	
LUNCH	
2 ounces dairy protein (list 4)	sandwich: 2 ounces skim milk
2 carbohydrates (list 3)	cheese, 2 slices bread
1/2 fat (list 5)	1/2 teaspoon margarine
1 1/2 vegetable (list 3)	1 1/2 cup fresh peas
list 1 vegetables as desired	large tomato salad with onion ring
1 fruit (list 2)	1 cup watermelon cubes
1 cup non-fat milk	1 cup non-fat milk
water	
MID-AFTERNOON	
1 fruit (list 2)	1 large tangerine
water	
DINNER	
2 ounces dairy protein or 1 egg (list 4)	1 egg omelet & 1 oz. lowfat cottage cheese
2 carbohydrates (list 3)	1 small baked potato
1 fat (list 5)	1 slice bread
2 vegetable (list 3)	1 teaspoon margarine
list 1 vegetables as desired	2/3 cup lentils
1 fruit (list 2)	large fresh spinach salad with
1 cup non-fat milk	chopped radishes and cucumbers
water	12 fresh grapes
	1 cup non-fat milk
BEDTIME	
1 cup non-fat milk	1 cup non-fat milk
1 carbohydrate (list 3)	4 melba toast

carbohydrate	225 gm	60% calories
protein	84 gm	22% calories
fat	30 gm	18% calories
cholesterol	<450 mg	
salt	<3.5 gm	

VEGETARIAN DIET 5
(1800 CALORIES)

Basic Diet Plan	Sample Menu
BREAKFAST	
1 fruit (list 2)	1/2 cup orange juice
2 carbohydrates (list 3)	1/2 cup oatmeal
	1 slice toast
1 fat (list 5)	1 teaspoon margarine
1 cup non-fat milk	1 cup non-fat milk
water	
MID-MORNING	
1 carbohydrate (list 3)	1 slice bread
1/2 fat (list 5)	1/2 teaspoon margarine
water	
LUNCH	
2 ounces dairy protein (list 4)	2 ounces cottage cheese
4 carbohydrates (list 3)	1 cup rice or beans
1 vegetable (list 3)	2 slices bread
1 fat (list 5)	1 cup Hubbard squash
list 1 vegetables as desired	1 teaspoon margarine
1 cup non-fat milk	large mixed green salad
water	1 cup non-fat milk
MID-AFTERNOON	
1 fruit (list 2)	1/2 cup pineapple chunks
1 carbohydrate (list 3)	4 soda crackers
water	
DINNER	
2 ounces dairy protein (list 4)	omelet: 1 egg, 1 ounce American cheese
3 carbohydrates (list 3)	1/2 cup steamed parsley rice
2 vegetable (list 3)	2 slices bread
list 1 vegetables as desired	2/3 cup corn
1 fruit (list 2)	lettuce and tomato salad
1 cup non-fat milk	1/2 cup sliced peaches
water	1 cup non-fat milk
BEDTIME	
1 fruit (list 2)	1 small apple

carbohydrate	286 gm	64% calories
protein	86 gm	19% calories
fat	33 gm	17% calories
cholesterol	<450 mg	
salt	<4.5 gm	

VEGETARIAN DIET 6
(2000 CALORIES)

Basic Diet Plan	Sample Menu
BREAKFAST	
1 fruit (list 2)	1/2 cup blended orange and grape-
3 carbohydrates (list 3)	fruit juice
1 fat (list 5)	2 slices toast
1 cup non-fat milk	1/2 cup farina
water	1 teaspoon margarine
	1 cup non-fat milk
MID-MORNING	
1 fruit (list 2)	1 small fresh pear
1 carbohydrate (list 3)	1 slice toast
water	
LUNCH	
3 ounces dairy protein (list 4)	3 ounces cottage cheese
4 carbohydrates (list 3)	1 cup beans or rice
1 fat (list 5)	2 slices bread
1 vegetable unit (list 3)	1 teaspoon margarine
list 1 vegetables as desired	1 cup steamed peas and carrots
1 cup non-fat milk	large tomato-cucumber salad
water	1 cup non-fat milk
MID-AFTERNOON	
1 fruit (list 2)	1/2 cup sliced peaches
1 carbohydrate (list 3)	4 unsalted crackers
water	
DINNER	
2 ounces dairy protein (list 4)	cheese omelet: 1 egg 1 ounce skim
4 carbohydrates (list 3)	milk cheese
2 vegetables (list 3)	1 large baked potato
list 1 vegetables as desired	2 slices bread
1 cup non-fat milk	1 cup carrots
water	mixed green salad
	1 cup non-fat milk
BEDTIME	
1 carbohydrate (list 3)	4 crackers
1 fruit (list 2)	1 small apple

carbohydrate	316 gm	64% calories
protein	97 mg	20% calories
fat	35 gm	16% calories
cholesterol	<450 mg	
salt	<5 gm	

Food Exchange List for All Diets

General Rules

1. Eat only foods listed on this diet, and in amounts indicated. Do not skip meals or feedings. Prepare and eat all food without added fat (oils, butter, margarine), sugar, salt or gravy.

2. Use fresh or frozen meats, fish, fruit, and vegetables.

3. Salt and sugar substitutes may be used with your doctor's approval. Drink at least 1 glass of water before or with each meal.

4. Learn the caloric value of everything you eat.

List 1

Miscellaneous very low calorie foods: 25 calories per serving or less.

Seasoning: cinnamon, garlic, lemon, dry mustard, mint, nutmeg, parsley, pepper, sugarless sweeteners, spices, vanilla, vinegar, low-sodium tomato juice.

Salad Dressing: vinegar, lemon, pepper, parsley, garlic, salt substitute, dry mustard, and other spices.

Other foods: cranberries, diet soft drinks, decaffeinated coffee, other coffee substitute (Postum, Breakfast Cup, Sanocaf).

Vegetables: asparagus, broccoli, brussels sprouts, cabbage, cauliflower, cucumber, eggplant, lettuce, mushrooms, peppers, radishes, string beans, summer squash, tomatoes, watercress, wax beans, celery.

List 2

Fruit: 50 calories per serving.

apple	1 (2″ dia.)
applesauce	1/2 cup
apricots	2 medium
banana	1 small
strawberries	1 cup
blueberries	2/3 cup
cantaloupe	1/4 (6″ dia.)
cherries	10 large
grapefruit	1/2 small
grapefruit juice	1/2 cup
grapes	12
grape juice	1/4 cup
honeydew	1/8 (7″)
mango	1/2 small
orange	1 small
orange juice	1/2 cup

peach	1 medium
pear	1 small
pineapple	1/2 cup
pineapple juice	1/3 cup
plums	2 medium
prune juice	1/4 cup
tangerine	1 large
watermelon	1 cup

List 3

Carbohydrate: 70 calories per serving

bread or tortilla	1 slice
roll	1 (2″ dia.)
crackers	4 unsalted
cereals, cooked	1/2 cup
dry	3/4 cup
rice, grits, cooked	1/2 cup
beans, lima, navy	1/2 cup
baked	1/4 cup
spaghetti, noodles, macaroni	1/2 cup
corn, lentils, split peas	1/3 cup
potato, white	1 (2″ dia.)
onions	1 cup
peas, green	1 cup
winter squash	1 cup
turnips, beets, rutabagas	1 cup
carrots	1 cup

List 4

Protein: 75 calories per serving

   Low fat cottage cheese: 1/4 cup (use 1 portion only daily). Non-fat milk, jello: 3/4 cup.

   Eggs: Limit eggs to 2–4 per week. On other days substitute 1/2 cup cooked cereal or 3/4 cup dry ceareal.

List 5

Fats: 45 calories per teaspoonful

   Use 1 teaspoon special margarine (first ingredient liquid oil, corn, safflower or soy), polyunsaturated cooking oil (corn or safflower), sauce or dressing made with corn or safflower oil.

12
Extra-Calorie Diets for Athletes and Heavy Laborers

Our studies, based on carefully maintained food diaries, have shown that 1000–2000 calories per day are adequate for maintaining optimal weight in the vast majority of relatively sedentary city dwellers. Under certain circumstances, however, a higher caloric level than this is indicated to achieve or maintain optimal weight and vigor. Those engaged in heavy physical labor, and certain types of athletes require greater nourishment. There is one qualification to this statement: These individuals should not be above optimal weight.

Typical High Risk Extra-Calorie Diets

Current ways of increasing calorie intake, whether advised by the athletic coach or trainer, physician, dietitian, or parent, are similar in theory and practice. All increase the amounts of the typical U.S. diet: meat, eggs, dairy products, bread products, and high carbohydrate-fat desserts. Such a diet increases the already excessively high animal-fat-cholesterol-sugar-salt-protein content of the usual U.S. diet. The net effect is to exaggerate the serious defects of the American diet.

The long-term results of this approach may be disastrous, for these individuals are subjected to an even greater risk of cardiovascular diseases than the average American adult whose risk is already very high. The habit of excess calorie intake developed during childhood and young adulthood becomes deeply ingrained. Too frequently, this eating pattern persists long after the need for extra calories exists, and when the neutralizing effect of increased physical activity is no longer present. In this setting, obesity, premature atherosclerosis, diabetes, and hypertension flourish with a high toll of heart attacks and strokes.

Synthetic Vitamin Supplements

Another popular part of the athlete's diet is the use of synthetic vitamins in large doses. Unless clearcut evidence of vitamin deficiency exists, the benefits derived from synthetic vitamins as supplements to the American diet are doubtful at best. The vitamin content of the American and Optimal Diets must be considered more than adequate because of the abundance of meat, vegetables, and fruit. The harmful effects of vitamin A and vitamin D overdosage are well documented in the medical literature. Detrimental effects of chronic overdosage of vitamins B, C, and E have not been established, but remain a possibility. Excess amounts of vitamin C may be harmful because they are excreted as ascorbic acid itself, dehydroascorbic acid, or oxalate. Increased oxalate in the urine may give rise to oxalate stones in the urinary tract. Oxalate stones are the most common type of renal stone in the U.S. Furthermore, acidification of the urine by large amounts of ascorbic acid and dehydroascorbic acid may precipitate uric acid and cystine stones in the urinary tract of predisposed patients (with gout, cystinuria, or chronic urinary infection).

Until the benefits of excessive dosage of a given vitamin for the individual when no clinical or laboratory evidence of deficiency are established, we do not recommend supplementation of the American or the Optimal Diet with synthetic vitamins. The supplementation of the athlete's diet with vitamins is even less justified.

Optimal Extra-Calorie Diet

Our technique for achieving optimal extra-calorie diets is to start with the 2000-calorie Optimal Diet and to increase its caloric level primarily by adding more vegetables, whole grain products, and fruit. Our extra-calorie diets are given at the end of this chapter.

It should be noted that they contain only a small increase in meat and a small increase in protein over the highest calorie Optimal Diet. This is to avoid excessive amounts of animal fat and protein. The dangers of animal fat are now well known. In contrast, it is widely believed that high protein intakes are desirable for athletes and some eat up to five times the minimal requirement. Actually, there is no evidence that extra physical exertion increases the requirement for protein. Furthermore, there is evidence that excessive amounts of dietary protein may be detrimental to the kidney, and to the arteries by causing the initial injury that leads to atherosclerosis.[60]

Carbohydrate "Loading" for Long-Distance Runners

There are many special diets advocated for athletes. To our knowledge none of these have been proved to augment performance in competiton. The popular carbohydrate "loading" or "packing" method proposed for long distance runners has recently been criticized on the grounds that overstuffing the muscle cells with glycogen may stiffen and weigh down the muscles too much for best performance and also destroy muscle cells.[61]

These diets are examples of the common fallacy that if a certain amount of a nutrient is essential, gobs of it should be much better. *We believe that any abnormal or unbalanced diet is more apt to have harmful effects on the body than to have a significant favorable effect on performance.* The paths to best performance in life and in athletics are optimal nutrition (the right nutrients in the right amounts) and sound training methods.

Nourishment Before and During Competition

There is much interest in which foods and beverages should be consumed just before and during athletic contests. Most authorities agree that the last full sized meal should be a minimum of four hours before competition to allow for complete emptying of the stomach.

As to nourishment during competition, opinions vary from complete fasting to small feedings high in protein or carbohydrates (e.g., amino acid tablets, candy, crackers, vitamins, etc.). Glucose and electrolyte solutions (ERG, Gatorade, etc.) have become popular as substitutes for the timehonored water bucket in order to restore sweat electrolytes and supply "quick energy."

Because most athletic contests (with such exceptions as the marathon and five sets of tennis) require sustained high activity for an hour or less, it is doubtful that the replacement of electrolytes or calories during the contest is a physiological necessity. Nonetheless, the beneficial effects of relieving thirst and hunger feeling should not be discounted. Water or any pleasant tasting beverage is acceptable as long as the quantity of it is kept *small at any one time* (one to four ounces) and fat is not present (to avoid abdominal fullness). Sugar content should be low enough to avoid dehydration (less than 2.5 percent). Therefore, we suggest plain water or a diluted orange juice-milk powder mixture. (One can of frozen orange juice concentrate mixed with water—add four to six tablespoons of dry skim-milk powder, according to taste, mix well in blender and dilute in half with water before use.) This drink can be very palatable, thirst-quenching, as well as relieve hunger feelings and excessive gastric acidity from nervous tension. Most beverages do not achieve all of these objectives.

EXTRA-CALORIE DIET 1
(2400 CALORIES)

Basic Diet Plan	Sample Menu
BREAKFAST	
2 fruit units (list 2)	1 cup orange juice
3 carbohydrate units (list 3)	1/2 cup oatmeal
1 egg 3x/wk.	2 slices toast
1 fat unit (list 5)	1 teaspoon margarine
1 cup non-fat milk	1 cup non-fat milk
beverage	coffee substitute
water	
MID-MORNING	
1 cup non-fat milk	1 cup non-fat milk
1 carbohydrate unit (list 3)	1 slice bread
water	
LUNCH	
2 oz. protein (list 4)	sandwich: 2 oz. skim milk cheese
4 carbohydrate units (list 3)	4 slices bread
1 fat unit (list 5)	1 teaspoon margarine
1 vegetable unit (list 3)	1 cup green peas
list 1 vegetables as desired	1 cup cole slaw with green pepper
1 fruit unit (list 2)	1 large tangerine
water	
MID-AFTERNOON	
1 fruit unit (list 2)	1 small apple
2 carbohydrate unit (list 3)	8 pieces melba toast
1 cup non-fat milk	1 cup non-fat milk
water	
DINNER	
3 oz. protein	3 oz. roast turkey
4 carbohydrate units (list 4)	1 cup steamed noodles
2 vegetables (list 3)	2 slices bread
list 1 vegetables as desired	2/3 cup corn
1 fat unit (list 5)	radishes and celery hearts
water	1 teaspoon margarine
BEDTIME	
1 fruit unit (list 2)	1/2 cup sliced peaches
1 carbohydrate unit (list 3)	4 soda crackers
1 cup non-fat milk	1 cup non-fat milk

carbohydrate	383 gm	64% calories
protein	116 gm	19% calories
fat	45 gm	17% calories
cholesterol	<200 mg	(no egg)
salt	<3.5 gm	

EXTRA-CALORIE DIET 2
(2700 CALORIES)

Basic Diet Plan	**Sample Menu**
BREAKFAST	
2 fruit units (list 2)	1 cup apricots
4 carbohydrate units (list 3)	1 cup oatmeal
1 egg 3x/wk.	2 slices toast
2 fat units (list 5)	2 teaspoons margarine
1 cup non-fat milk	1 cup non-fat milk
beverage	coffee substitute
water	
MID-MORNING	
1 fruit unit (list 2)	1/2 cup applesauce
2 carbohydrate units (list 3)	2 slices toast
water	
LUNCH	
2 oz. protein (list 4)	2 oz. tuna
5 carbohydrate units (list 3)	2 cups noodles
1 fat unit (list 5)	2 slices bread
1 vegetable unit (list 3)	1 teaspoon margarine
list 1 vegetables as desired	1 cup green peas
1 cup non-fat milk	lettuce and tomato salad
water	1 sliced banana
	1 cup non-fat milk
MID-AFTERNOON	
1 fruit unit (list 2)	1/2 cup fresh fruit compote
2 carbohydrate units (list 3)	8 pieces melba toast
water	
DINNER	
3 oz. protein (list 4)	3 oz. broiled chicken
4 carbohydrate units (list 3)	1 cup mashed potato
2 vegetables (list 3)	2 slices bread
1 fat unit (list 5)	2/3 cup corn or lentils
1 vegetable as desired	1 teaspoon margarine
1 fruit unit (list 2)	radish roses and celery hearts
1 cup non-fat milk	1 cup fresh strawberries
water	1 cup non-fat milk
BEDTIME	
1 fruit (list 2)	1 large tangerine
2 carbohydrate units (list 3)	8 soda crackers
1 cup non-fat milk	1 cup non-fat milk

carbohydrate	438 gm	65% calories
protein	124 gm	18% calories
fat	50 gm	17% calories
cholesterol	<200 mg	(no egg)
salt	<5 gm	

EXTRA-CALORIE DIET 3
(3000 CALORIES)

Basic Diet Plan	Sample Menu
BREAKFAST	
1 fruit unit (list 2)	1/2 cup orange juice
3 eggs per week	1 cup farina
4 carbohydrate units (list 3)	2 slices toast
1 fat unit (list 5)	1 teaspoon margarine
1 cup non-fat milk	1 cup non-fat milk
beverage	coffee substitute
water	
MID-MORNING	
1 fruit unit (list 2)	1 small pear
3 carbohydrate units (list 3)	3 slices toast
1 cup non-fat milk	1 cup non-fat milk
water	
LUNCH	
1 fruit unit (list 2)	1/2 cup sliced peaches
2 ounces protein (list 4)	2 ounces salmon
5 carbohydrate units (list 3)	1-1/2 cup steamed noodles
1 fat unit (list 5)	2 slices bread
1 vegetable unit (list 3)	1 teaspoon margarine
list 1 vegetables as desired	1 cup green peas
water	sliced tomato salad with lemon
MID-AFTERNOON	
1 fruit unit (list 2)	1/2 sliced banana
4 carbohydrate units (list 3)	16 soda crackers
DINNER	
3 ounces protein (list 4)	3 ounces lean ground veal
4 carbohydrate units (list 3)	1 medium baked potato (8 oz.)
1 fat unit (list 5)	2 slices bread
2 vegetable units (list 3)	1 teaspoon margarine
list 1 vegetables as desired	2/3 cup lentils
	cucumber and endive salad
BEDTIME	
1 fruit unit (list 2)	1 small fresh pear
3 carbohydrate units (list 3)	12 pieces melba toast
1 cup non-fat milk	1 cup non-fat milk
1 fat unit (list 5)	1 teaspoon margarine

carbohydrate	488 gm	65% calories
protein	136 gm	18% calories
fat	50 gm	15% calories
cholesterol	<250 mg	(no egg)
salt	<4.5 gm	

Food Exchange List for All Diets

GENERAL RULES

1. Eat only foods listed on this diet, and in amounts indicated. Do not skip meals or feedings. Prepare and eat all food without added fat, sugar, salt, or gravy.

2. Use fresh or frozen meats, fish, fruit, and vegetables.

3. Salt and sugar substitutes may be used with your doctor's approval. Drink at least 1 glass of water before or with each meal.

4. Learn the caloric value of everything you eat.

LIST 1

Miscellaneous very low calorie foods: 25 calories per serving or less.

Seasoning: cinnamon, garlic, lemon, dry mustard, mint, nutmeg, parsley, pepper, sugarless sweeteners, spices, vanilla, vinegar, low-sodium tomato juice.

Salad Dressing: vinegar, lemon, pepper, parsley, garlic, salt substitute, dry mustard, garlic and other spices.

Other foods: cranberries, diet soft drinks, decaffeinated coffee, coffee substitute.

Vegetables: asparagus, broccoli, brussels sprouts, cabbage, cauliflower, cucumber, eggplant, lettuce, mushrooms, peppers, radishes, string beans, summer squash, tomatoes, watercress, wax beans, celery.

List 2

Fruit: 50 calories per serving

apple	1 (2" dia.)
applesauce	1/2 cup
apricots	2 medium
banana	1 small
strawberries	1 cup
blueberries	2/3 cup
cantaloupe	1/4 (6" dia.)
cherries	10 large
grapefruit	1/2 small
grapefruit juice	1/2 cup
grapes	12
watermelon	1 cup
grape juice	1/4 cup
honeydew	1/8 (7")
mango	1/2 small
orange	1 small
orange juice	1/2 cup

peach	1 medium
pear	1 small
pineapple	1/2 cup
pineapple juice	1/3 cup
plums	2 medium
prune juice	1/4 cup
tangerine	1 large

List 3

Carbohydrate: 70 calories per serving

bread or tortilla	1 slice
roll	1 (2" dia.)
crackers	4 unsalted
cereals, cooked	1/2 cup
dry	3/4 cup
rice, grits, cooked	1/2 cup
beans, lima, navy	1/2 cup
baked	1/4 cup
spaghetti, noodles, macaroni	1/2 cup
corn, lentils, split peas	1/3 cup
potato, white	1 (2" dia.)
onions	1 cup
peas, green	1 cup
winter squash	1 cup
turnips, beets, rutabagas	1 cup
carrots	1 cup

List 4

Protein: 75 calories per serving

Meat: turkey, chicken, veal, lamb, beef: 1 slice (3" x 2" x 1/8" or 1 ounce). *Fish:* bass, bluefish, catfish, cod, flounder, halibut, rockfish, salmon, sole, tuna (fresh, canned in water, or washed with water—same amount as meat).

Low-fat cottage cheese: 1/4 cup (use 1 portion only daily). Non-fat milk, jello: 3/4 cup.

Eggs: Limit eggs to 2–4 per week. On other days substitute 1/2 cup cooked cereal or 3/4 cup dry cereal.

Most desirable eat others only 1–3 times per week.

List 5

Fats: 45 calories per teaspoonful

Use 1 teaspoon special margarine (first ingredient liquid oil, corn, safflower, or soy), polyunsaturated cooking oil (corn or safflower), sauce or dressing made with corn or safflower oil.

Part Four:
Diet and Disease

13
Introduction

The relationship between daily eating habits (diet) and the major diseases of the U.S. and other industrial nations of the world is shown in Fig. 13–1. Scientific evidence indicates that diet plays a major role in causing these common and disabling (or fatal) diseases. Furthermore, the evidence that these diseases can be prevented or controlled by relatively simple changes in eating habits is convincing enough to advise their use without further delay. The Optimal Diets described in Chapter 10 were designed specifically to prevent or control these diseases. In some instances, modifications of the basic Optimal Diet is necessary to achieve maximal effectiveness. In the following chapters the dietary treatment of these important and common diseases will be described in greater detail. The relationship of diet to heart disease has been discussed in Chapter 10.

Obesity, hypertension, hyperlipoproteinemia, diabetes, cancer, and cirrhosis are extremely common diseases in the U.S.: Many millions suffer from one or more of these disorders. In the early stages of these diseases, there are no symptoms and the people feel entirely well. For example, several surveys have shown that at least 50% of people with high blood pressure do not know they have it.[62]

At this stage (before complications develop), these individuals have the potential of controlling their diseases and achieving optimal health-fitness. Optimal living habits can be very effective in preventing the usual complications. It is precisely in the early stages of these diseases that the medical profession has failed to act positively and energetically. The physician has not been trained in the use of diet and exercise therapy, and seldom emphasizes it before the disease reaches the stage of symptoms and complications. At this late stage other forms of therapy become necessary and the chances of achieving optimal health-fitness diminish considerably.

Nonetheless, even in these individuals, changes in eating habits and other living habits may still substantially improve health-fitness.

Figure 13–1

RELATIONSHIP BETWEEN DIET AND DISEASE

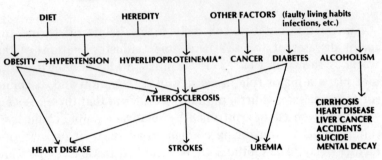

*high blood cholesteral and triglycerides

14
Obesity
(Overweight)

Obesity is a complex, confused subject: an ill-defined disorder about which countless articles and books have been written by a wide variety of "authorities." It is the object of universal and highly emotional interest to people of all ages and in all walks of life. Many false ideas on the subject are spread by both laymen and physicians and often defended with strong conviction. Enormous amounts of money are spent by the public on weight reduction treatment offered by "therapists": lay organizations, medical cultists, physicians who specialize in weight reduction, as well as physicians in general or specialty practice. Despite much experimentation work and some attractive theories, solid evidence on many aspects of the subject is meager, and a surprising number of misconceptions about it remain widespread.

Traditional U.S. Treatment

The need for more effective therapy for obesity is made obvious by the extremely high incidence of it in the United States, and the extremely low percentage of success in its treatment. It has been variously estimated to occur in 40 to 90% of the adult population, depending on whether standards of "normal," "desirable," or "optimal" are employed. The number of persons who achieve a significant weight reduction and maintain this reduction for a year or more is very low (less than 5%).

We believe that these poor results are due in large measure to: (a) emphasis on one phase of the treatment only (usually caloric intake), (b) failure to tailor the regimen to the individual, or (c) the "crash" program philosophy of therapy (reliance on medications, short-term diets, and environments like spas or weight-control camps).

151

These so-called aids to weight reduction are not only unsuccessful, but actually aggravate the disorder by delaying the effective treatment, by lowering self-confidence, by establishing dependence, and by directing efforts away from the establishment of optimal living habits.

Optimal Prevention and Treatment Program

Our therapeutic program is based on the following principles:

• Obesity is a chronic, lifelong disorder that threatens all inhabitants of the U.S. and other highly developed countries because of the living habits characteristic of these countries.

• The criteria of successful therapy (or prevention) of this disorder is the achievement and lifelong maintenance of an optimal weight.

• Treatment must emphasize the development of optimal living and eating habits and must be designed for lifelong suitability for each individual.

Weight Reduction Diets

The weight reduction diets included in this chapter range between 90 and 860 calories per day. The situations in which these may be appropriate are described briefly. (Diets of higher calorie value for weight reduction or weight maintenance are described in chapter 10, Optimal Diet.) Differences between individuals are so great that one must estimate a caloric requirement that will achieve a reduction of 1 to 2 pounds per week. Try it, then shift to a higher or lower calorie diet according to weight loss results.

The programs of physical activity described in earlier chapters are appropriate to weight control, with the precaution that excess weight may impose additional strain on the musculoskeletal system. For this reason certain principles of physical conditioning (Chapter 7) used as gradual progression, duration, and intensity of the exercise should be carefully followed.

The eating patterns that lead to obesity are habits typically established early in life. Permanent changes in weight, then, will require permanent changes in eating habits: food preparation, food selection, and the manner in which we eat.

It is important to obtain professional medical help to detect and treat the disorders commonly associated with obesity, i.e., hypertension, diabetes, heart disease and hyperlipoproteinemias (excessive blood cholesterol and triglycerides).

We define successful treatment of obesity as achieving and maintaining optimal weight for at least one year. Anything less than this goal will almost invariably result in a recurrence of obesity.

We have found that the successful type of diet is generally correlated with the degree of obesity, its duration, and the degree of physical activity of the patient. Therefore, we have developed diets of various caloric levels to be used according to the degree of overweight and level of physical activity. The diets are designed to be similar to and include the optimal diets described in Chapter 13. Described below are four caloric levels, all of which are closely related in structure, differing only in the quantities used.

Obesity Diet 1 (50–100 calories). This diet is used only in the hospital under close medical supervision. It is designed for persons with the most extreme degree of obesity (more than 100 pounds over optimal weight), who have shown an inadequate response to outpatient treatment with the usual low-calorie diet, etc., or for those who require more rapid weight reduction. It has been proved more acceptable with fewer side effects than the starvation diet (no calories) while resulting in a similar rate of weight loss (average one pound per day). As with the starvation diet a high fluid intake (over 3 quarts/day) must be maintained.

Obesity Diet 2 (350 calories). This diet is used for the extremely obese people following a weight loss of 20–25 pounds on the 90-calorie diet. It may be used on an out-patient basis for a short period (less than 1 month) under close medical supervision.

Obesity Diet 3 (580 calories). This diet is used for individuals who are 50–100 pounds over optimal weight, and who have low physical activity. It is recommended for short term use (less than 2 months) and under medical supervision.

Obesity Diet 4 (860 calories). This diet is used for patients who are less than 35 pounds over optimal weight and are moderately to very active.

Patients are moved from one calorie level to another depending on their progress. The goal is to reach a maintenance calorie level after optimal weight is arrived at. As soon as the patient achieves optimal weight, his diet is increased by 200–300 calories to prevent further loss of weight. If after several weeks of this diet, the weight remains unchanged or falls, it is increased again by the same number of calories and this process is continued until the patient begins to increase his weight above the optimal level. The maintenance caloric intake is arrived at when the patient takes the minimum number of calories necessary to maintain optimal weight and body fat.

Our experience indicates that the optimal maintenance caloric level for the vast majority of adult Americans (sedentary lifestyle) is between 1000 and 2000 calories, regardless of the age or sex. This is considerably below the caloric levels (2300–3300) recommended by the National Research Council and other nutritional authorities.

Because all of our diets have the same structure, it has been easy to go from one to the other without retraining the patient in eating habits or tastes. The diets are all designed for lifelong use from the standpoint of acceptability, content of essential food elements, economy, and variety.

The obesity diets in this chapter are similar to our diabetic and optimal diets, keeping with our concept that therapeutic diets should imitate the optimal diet whenever possible. Selecting a diet for a given patient depends on the caloric level indicated by body weight (in relation to individual optimal weight), percent body fat, and the actual response of body weight and fat to a trial of different caloric levels.

We believe that the widely recommended practice of establishing caloric intake based on a certain number of calories per pound of body weight is unrealistic. It ignores factors such as muscle and bone mass, which influence body weight in the individual and cannot be precalculated by any formula. Furthermore, it does not take into account the wide individual differences in energy expenditure for each physical activity. In the final analysis individual caloric requirements can only be arrived at by trial and error.

OBESITY DIET 1 (50–100 CALORIES)

This diet is used primarily in extreme cases of obesity. The patient is hospitalized under the supervision of a physician, who has knowledge of the effects of starvation therapy. Daily vitamin and mineral supplements must be added. No salt or sugar is given. All such patients must drink a minimum of 12 glasses of fluid each day (water, diet soft drink, coffee-like drink).

Basic Diet Plan	Sample Menu A	Sample Menu B
BREAKFAST		
1 cup salt-free, fat-free bouillon or broth 1 serving fresh or unsweetened canned fruit or juice calorie-free beverage water	1 cup salt-free, fat-free chicken broth 1/2 cup grapefruit sections coffee or tea with lemon and/or saccharin	1 cup salt-free, fat-free beef broth 1/2 cup orange juice coffee or tea with lemon and/or saccharin
MID-MORNING		
5 ounces diet gelatin calorie-free beverage water	5 ounces diet lime gelatin diet lemonade	5 ounces diet lemon gelatin diet soft drink
LUNCH		
1/2–1 ounce protein 1 cup green greens or List 1 vegetable calorie-free beverage water	2 tbsp. lowfat cottage cheese 4 large romaine leaves 2 tomato wedges 3 dietetic asparagus spears 2 radishes hot or iced tea with lemon	1 ounce shredded chicken 1/2 cup shredded lettuce 1 slice onion 2 large green pepper rings 2 large slices tomato hot spiced tea with lemon
MID-AFTERNOON		
calorie-free beverage water	diet soft drink	diet lemonade
DINNER		
1 cup salt-free, fat-free broth or consomme 2 low-calorie wafers 1 cup mixed green salad or List 1 vegetables with calorie-free dressing 5 ounces diet gelatin calorie-free beverage water	1 cup salt-free, fat-free beef consomme 2 low-calorie wheat wafers 1 cup shredded cabbage and green pepper slaw with vinegar dressing 5 ounces diet lemon gelatin hot tea or coffee substitute	1 cup salt-free, fat-free turkey broth 2 low-calorie wheat wafers 1 cup endive, escarole, and cucumber salad with tomato juice dressing 5 ounces diet orange gelatin hot tea or coffee substitute
BEDTIME		
5 ounces diet gelatin calorie-free beverage	5 ounces diet pineapple gelatin diet lemonade	5 ounces diet raspberry gelatin diet soft drink

salt <100 mg

OBESITY DIET 2 (350 CALORIES)

Basic Diet Plan	Sample Menu A	Sample Menu B
BREAKFAST 1 fruit (list 2) 1/2 carbohydrate (list 3) 1/2 cup skim milk coffee substitute water	1/2 small grapefruit 1/2 slice toast 1/2 cup skim milk coffee substitute	1/2 cup unsweetened applesauce 1/2 slice toast 1/2 cup skim milk coffee substitute
MID-MORNING 12 ounces diet drink water	12 ounces diet lemonade	12 ounces iced tea/ lemon
LUNCH 1 ounce protein (list 4) 1 cup vegetable (list 1) 1/2 cup skim milk beverage water	1 ounce white chicken 1 cup mixed green salad with tomato/ vinegar 1/2 cup skim milk coffee substitute	1/4 cup cottage cheese 1 large sliced tomato on 2 large lettuce leaves 1/2 cup skim milk coffee substitute
MID-AFTERNOON 12 ounces diet drink water	12 ounces diet soft drink	12 ounces diet lemonade
DINNER 1 ounce protein (list 4) 1 cup vegetable (list 1) 1 diet gelatin or 1 fruit (list 2) beverage water	1 ounce lean roast beef 1 cup asparagus spears 3/4 cup diet lime gelatin coffee substitute	1 ounce broiled white fish 1 cup fresh broccoli 1 fresh tangerine coffee substitute
BEDTIME 12 ounces diet drink	12 ounces iced tea/ lemon	12 ounces diet soft drink
carbohydrate protein fat cholesterol salt	40 gm 23 gm 12 gm <150 mg <0.5 gm	45% calories 25% calories 30% calories

OBESITY DIET 3 (580 CALORIES)

Basic Diet Plan	Sample Menu A	Sample Menu B
BREAKFAST 1 fruit (list 2) 1/2 carbohydrate (list 3) 1/2 cup non-fat milk coffee or tea water	1/2 cup orange juice 1/2 slice toast 1/2 cup non-fat milk coffee or tea	1/4 (6") cantaloupe 1/2 slice toast 1/2 cup non-fat milk coffee or tea
MID-MORNING 12 ounces diet drink water	12 ounces diet lemonade	12 ounces diet soft drink
LUNCH 1 ounce protein (list 4) 1 cup vegetable (list 1) 1/2 carbohydrate (list 3) 1 teaspoon fat (list 5) 1/2 cup non-fat milk beverage water	1 ounce sliced turkey 1 cup lettuce & tomato salad/vinegar dressing 1/2 slice bread 1 teaspoon special margarine 1/2 cup non-fat milk coffee substitute	1/4 cup cottage cheese 1 cup cucumber, radish, & shredded cabbage/vinegar dressing 1/2 slice bread 1 teaspoon special margarine 1/2 cup non-fat milk coffee substitute
MID-AFTERNOON 12 ounces diet drink water	12 ounces coffee substitute	12 ounces diet lemonade
DINNER 1 ounce protein (list 4) 1 cup vegetable (list 1) 1/2 carbohydrate (list 3) 1 teaspoon fat (list 5) 1 fruit (list 2) beverage water	1 ounce ground beef 1 cup fresh cauliflower 1/2 slice bread 1 teaspoon special margarine 1 cup cubed watermelon coffee substitute	1 ounce baked fish/lemon 1 cup fresh asparagus 1/2 slice bread 1 teaspoon special margarine 1/2 cup applesauce coffee substitute
BEDTIME 12 ounces diet drink	12 ounces diet soft drink	12 ounces coffee substitute
carbohydrate protein fat cholesterol salt	59 gm 25 gm 22 gm <150 mg <1.25 gm	50% calories 17% calories 33% calories

OBESITY DIET 4A (860 CALORIES)

Two plans are shown for the 860 calorie diet. For the person who feels that he can best follow a diet that allows some basic protein in *each* meal, Obesity Diet 4A is given. For the individual who prefers most of his protein in the evening meal, with a "bulky" low-carbohydrate lunch, Obesity Diet 4B is given.

Basic Diet Plan	Sample Menu A	Sample Menu B
BREAKFAST		
1 fruit (list 2)	1/2 grapefruit	1/2 small banana
1/2 slice bread	1/2 slice bread	1/2 slice toast
1/2 cup non-fat milk	1/2 cup non-fat milk	1/2 cup oatmeal
1 egg or egg substitute	1 egg	1/2 cup non-fat milk
coffee substitute	coffee substitute	coffee substitute
water		
MID-MORNING		
12 ounces diet drink	12 ounces lemonade	12 ounces iced tea/
water		lemon
LUNCH		
2 ounces protein (list 4)	1/2 cup tuna	1/2 cup cottage
1 cup vegetable (list 1)	1 cup tomato, cucum-	cheese
1/2 vegetable (list 3)	ber, & romaine salad	1 cup cole slaw with
1/2 slice bread	1/2 cup carrot sticks	green pepper
1/2 teaspoon fat (list 5)	1/2 slice bread	1/2 cup carrot sticks
1 fruit (list 2)	1/2 teaspoon special	1/2 slice bread
1/2 cup non-fat milk	margarine	1/2 teaspoon special
beverage	1 large tangerine	margarine
water	1/2 cup non-fat milk	1 small fresh pear
	coffee substitute	1/2 cup non-fat milk
		coffee substitute
MID-AFTERNOON		
12 ounces diet drink	12 ounces iced tea/	12 ounces diet
water	lemon	lemonade
DINNER		
2 ounces protein (list 4)	2 ounces lean roast beef	2 ounces broiled fish
1 cup vegetable (list 1)	1 cup brussels sprouts	1 cup fresh string
1/2 vegetable (list 3)	1/2 cup peas	beans
1 slice bread	1 slice bread	1/2 cup winter
1/2 teaspoon fat (list 5)	1/2 teaspoon special	squash
1 fruit (list 2)	margarine	1 slice bread
1/2 cup non-fat milk	1/2 cup applesauce	1/2 teaspoon special
beverage	1/2 cup non-fat milk	margarine
water	coffee substitute	1/2 cup orange
		sections
		1/2 cup non-fat milk
		coffee substitute
BEDTIME		
12 ounces diet drink	12 ounces diet soft	12 ounces diet soft
	drink	drink
carbohydrate	93 gm	43% calories
protein	55 gm	26% calories
fat	30 gm	31% calories
cholesterol	<200 mg	(without egg)
salt	<2 gm	

OBESITY DIET 4B (860 CALORIES)

Basic Diet Plan	Sample Menu

BREAKFAST

1 fruit (list 2)   1/2 small grapefruit
1 carbohydrate (list 3) *or* 1 egg*   1 slice toast
  or egg substitute   1/2 teaspoon margarine
1/2 fat (list 5)   1/2 cup non-fat milk
1/2 cup non-fat milk   coffee substitute
12 ounces low calorie drink**
water

MID-MORNING

1/2 carbohydrate (list 3)   1/2 slice toast
12 ounces low calorie drink   12 ounces diet lemonade

LUNCH

2 cooked (or raw) vegetables (list 1)   1 cup cooked broccoli with lemon
1 salad with low calorie dressing   1 cup stewed tomatoes with dill
  (list 1)   seasoning
1/2 vegetable (list 3)   1 cup mixed vegetable salad with
1 fruit (list 2)   vinegar dressing
12 ounces low calorie drink   1 cup watermelon
water   12 ounces coffee substitute

MID-AFTERNOON

1/2 cup non-fat milk (or 5 oz. diet   1/2 cup non-fat milk *or* 5 oz. diet
  gelatin)   gelatin
1/2 carbohydrate (list 3)   1/2 slice bread
12 ounces low calorie drink   12 ounces diet soft drink

DINNER

4 protein (list 4)   4 ounces broiled chicken
1/2 carbohydrate (list 3)   1/4 cup steamed rice
1/2 fat (list 5)   1/2 teaspoon margarine
1 salad with low calorie dressing   1 cup cucumber-tomato salad with
  (list 1)   diet dressing
2 vegetables (list 1)   1 cup zucchini
12 ounces low calorie drink   1 cup mushrooms
water   12 ounces coffee substitute

BEDTIME

1/2 cup non-fat milk   1/2 cup non-fat milk
1 fruit (list 2)   1 tangerine
12 ounces low calorie drink   12 ounces diet soft drink

carbohydrate	92 gm	43% calories
protein	56 gm	25% calories
fat	30 gm	32% calories
cholesterol	<200 mg	(without egg)
salt	<2 gm	

*Two times weekly.
**Sano-caf, Breakfast Cup, tea, water, diet lemonade, diet soft drink, salt-free tomato juice, Postum.

Food Exchange List for All Diets

General Rules

1. Eat only foods listed on this diet, and in amounts indicated. Do not skip meals or feedings. Prepare and eat all food without added fat, sugar, salt, or gravy.

2. Use fresh or frozen meats, fish, vegetables, and fruit.

3. Salt and sugar substitutes may be used with your doctor's approval. Drink at least 1 glass of water before or with each meal and snack.

4. Learn the caloric value of everything you eat.

List 1

Miscellaneous very low calorie foods: 25 calories per serving or less.

Seasoning: cinnamon, garlic, lemon, dry mustard, mint, nutmeg, parsley, pepper, sugarless sweeteners, spices, vanilla, vinegar, low sodium tomato juice.

Salad Dressing: vinegar, lemon, pepper, parsley, garlic, salt substitute, dry mustard, and other spices.

Other foods: cranberries, diet soft drinks, decaffeinated coffee, postum.

Vegetables: asparagus, broccoli, brussels sprouts, cabbage, cauliflower, cucumber, eggplant, lettuce, mushrooms, peppers, radishes, string beans, summer squash, tomatoes, watercress, wax beans, celery.

List 2

Fruit: 50 calories per serving

apple	1 (2" dia.)
applesauce	1/2 cup
apricots	2 medium
banana	1 small
strawberries	1 cup
blueberries	2/3 cup
cantaloupe	1/4 (6" dia.)
cherries	10 large
grapefruit	1/2 small
grapefruit juice	1/2 cup
grapes	12
grape juice	1/4 cup
honeydew	1/8 (7")
mango	1/2 small
orange	1 small
orange juice	1/2 cup
peach	1 medium
pear	1 small
pineapple	1/2 cup

pineapple juice	1/3 cup
plums	2 medium
prune juice	1/4 cup
tangerine	1 large
watermelon	1 cup

List 3

Carbohydrate: 70 calories per serving

bread or tortilla	1 slice
roll	1 (2" dia.)
crackers	4 unsalted
cereals, cooked	1/2 cup
dry	3/4 cup
winter squash	1 cup
turnips, beets, rutabagas	1 cup
carrots	1 cup
potato, white	1 (2" dia.)
onions	1 cup
peas, green	1 cup
rice, grits, cooked	1/2 cup
beans, lima, navy	1/2 cup
baked	1/4 cup
spaghetti, noodles, macaroni	1/2 cup
corn, lentils, split peas	1/3 cup

List 4

Protein: 75 calories per serving

Meat: turkey, chicken, veal, lamb, beef: 1 slice (3" x 2" x 1/8" or 1 ounce) *Fish:* bass, bluefish, catfish, cod, flounder, halibut, rockfish, salmon, sole, tuna (fresh, canned in water, or washed with water): same amount as meat.

Low fat cottage cheese: 1/4 cup (use 1 portion only daily). Non-fat milk, jello: 3/4 cup

Eggs: Limit eggs to 2 per week. On other days substitute 1/2 cup cooked cereal or 3/4 cup dry cereal.

Fish and fowl are most desirable. Eat others only 1–2 times per week.

List 5

Fats: 45 calories per teaspoonful

Use 1 teaspoon special margarine (first ingredient liquid oil, corn, safflower or soy)), polyunsaturated cooking oil, (corn or safflower) sauce or dressing made with corn or safflower oil.

Weight Control Tips

1. Eat slowly and you will be satisfied with less food. Cut your food into small portions, take small mouthfuls and chew

slowly before swallowing. Sip beverage slowly, and it will seem like more.

2. Don't eat unless you're hungry. Before eating ask yourself if you are really hungry and don't eat unless you are. At meals, stop eating as soon as your hunger stops.

3. Put less food on your plate; you will be less tempted to eat more than is necessary to satisfy your hunger.

4. Drink a glass of water, tea, coffee, or other low-calorie beverage before each meal. Drink additional fluid during the meal; each swallow helps to fill you up and decreases hunger so that you are satisfied with less.

5. Omit salt or use it sparingly. Salt causes water retention, thereby increases your weight. In addition, it encourages you to eat more. It also raises blood pressure.

6. Avoid sugar in your beverages and food. A teaspoonful equals approximately 20 calories.

7. Use salads frequently. Ten large leaves of lettuce contain only 25 calories, and vegetables used in salads are equally low in calories. Tossed salad with a noncaloric dressing is a very satisfying snack or part of a meal.

8. Don't use butter, margarine, cream, fats, mayonnaise, or rich dressings. Two pats of butter with each meal equal 200 calories. Two tablespoons of mayonnaise in a salad are over 200 calories. Two tablespoons of cream in coffee 4 times a day equal nearly 300 calories.

9. Cut down on 2 or 3 items you won't miss. These small calorie savings daily save many pounds over the course of a year. If you eliminate 150 calories per day, which amounts to only 1 slice of bread and butter, a highball, and 1 tablespoon of rich salad dressing, you will lose 16 pounds a year. This technique is a simple form of reducing that is relatively painless. Not adhering to the above procedure explains why many people slowly gain weight over the years without realizing it.

10. If you are tempted to eat a high caloric food, taste a small amount, but do not eat the full portion.

11. Do not hesitate to tell your hostess or friends at a dinner that you are on a diet, and are not allowed to eat certain foods and must have small portions of the others.

12. Never take second helpings; be firm but polite and say

you are on a strict diet. Whenever it is not impolite, don't linger at the table and be tempted to take more food.

13. Try sugarless chewing gum or candy if tempted to take a between-meal snack.

14. Keep a calorie diary. In this way you can keep track of the number of calories you have consumed during the day, and it will remind you to stop eating when you have reached your limit.

15. Make a list of the zero-calorie items and learn them. In this way you can frequently satisfy your hunger without increasing your caloric intake. Have them at all times in your home.

16. Learn to use the low-calorie dairy products: nonfat milk and low-fat yogurt. These are high in protein and low in fat and calories; thus, they constitute ideal foods.

17. Take a picture of yourself in a bathing suit before you start dieting. This will prove helpful in spurring you on to your goal and will show you how much you have accomplished when you reach it.

18. A reward system is often helpful. For example, every time you are tempted to have a high caloric snack put the money it would cost into a special fund. When you have accumulated enough, buy yourself something that ordinarily would have been an extravagance.

19. Increase the level of your activity throughout the day and sleep less. Don't spend more than 7 hours in bed. You use up more than twice as many more calories out of bed than in bed.

20. Learn the low-calorie vegetables and eat them in quantity. These are: asparagus, bean sprouts, beet greens, broccoli, cabbage, cauliflower, celery, chard, cucumbers, endive, green beans, kale, lettuce, mushrooms, parsley, pimentos, green peppers, radishes, sauerkraut, spinach, summer squash, tomatoes, and watercress.

21. If possible, diet along with another overweight friend or spouse. You can compare weight losses and check each other to stay in line. You may even have a betting system whereby the one who breaks the diets pays a penalty.

22. Use low-calorie seasoning to spice up your meals. For example: fresh lemon juice, parsley, monosodium glutamate,

various salt substitutes, mint leaf, garlic, and vinegar, oregano, thyme, dill, bay leaves, pepper, chili peppers.

23. Keep your refrigerator filled with low-calorie foods and snacks in case you have an overwhelming temptation to eat between meals.

24. Guard against unscientific notions about food and dieting. These myths are handed down from generation to generation or from self-appointed nutrition experts. They are often costly, unrealistic, and harmful to your health.

25. Successful weight reduction depends on counting calories. You have to learn the caloric value of all the foods you eat. Healthy dieting depends on an intake of a well-balanced, low-calorie diet. A diet composed of 1, 2, or 3 foods does not satisfy these requirements, and therefore cannot be used over a long period of time.

26. Reduce the appetite by having a low-calorie snack of fruit or salad shortly before sitting down to the regular meal.

27. Don't be impatient with your progress. It takes time to lose weight and it should not be done too quickly. This gives your body a chance to adjust itself to its new size, and the stomach has an opportunity to shrink.

28. You might find that your friends make it more difficult for you to follow your reduction program. Their reasons for doing so are complex. Nearly all people dislike the unfamiliar and resist the possibility of any change of friends. They will tell you that you look better with more weight, that your disposition is better, and in other ways try to convince you that you will be happier and healthier the way you are. But remember, your first duty is to yourself. You have to be with yourself all the time, and you should strive to be a self you admire and want to be, not what others think is right for you.

29. Remember that when you reach your goal of the optimal weight your job is not over. Having been formerly overweight is something like being a former alcoholic. The fat is gone but your sensitivity to gaining weight will always exist. The scale will always be your most reliable instrument in determining your success and danger of potential failure. Watch it consistently, heed its warning, and you will never get back into serious trouble. Eventually you will become so stabilized in

your weight that there will be practically no weight fluctuations at all.

30. Increase your daily physical activity by the following measures:

(a) Do not remain in bed more than 7 hours per 24 hours.

(b) Reduce the amount of sitting you do to a minimum.

(c) Use the stairs, not the elevator.

(d) Be in a hurry when you walk.

(e) Walk more, ride less.

(f) Take a brisk, uninterrupted walk daily: start with 5–10 minutes, and gradually increase it to at least 30 minutes, preferably 1 hour.

15
Hypertension (High Blood Pressure)

Hypertension should concern all of us because it is so common and is one of the primary factors in the development of heart disease and strokes. Heredity factors may be involved, or it may result from a number of faulty living habits. A common cause is susceptibility to high salt intake.[63] It has been estimated that over 40% of Americans are genetically susceptible to hypertension, and more than twenty percent have it. Of those who have it, less than 50 percent know that they have it, and perhaps only ten percent of those who have it are getting adequate treatment.

Hypertension and Salt Intake

In those who are susceptible, salt intake has an appreciable impact on the development of hypertension. Populations eating about one to two grams of salt per day (Eskimos, Greenlanders, aboriginal Australians) have a very low incidence of high blood pressure. Americans average 10 to 20 grams of salt per day and have at least a twenty percent incidence. The northern Honshu of Japan consume 26 grams of salt per day and have an incidence of hypertension that is approximately 40 percent. Because there is a considerable amount of salt naturally in most foodstuffs, avoid (1) adding salt to food, and (2) using canned and packaged food, to which salt is typically added in large amounts. These precautions are especially important if there is a history of hypertension in the family.

Diet and Drug Therapy

Before the advent of modern anti-hypertensive drugs, diet therapy was the only effective way of controlling high blood pressure. Diet therapy was directed at the control of the frequently accompanying disorders: heart and kidney failure, obesity, and edema. Thus, the diets were low in sodium, protein, and/or calories; e.g., the Kempner rice diet. Diet therapy was limited by the monotony and relatively unpalatable nature of effective diets and the difficulty of obtaining long-term patient cooperation.

During the past decade a large number of new food products have made it possible to design more palatable diets, nearly unlimited in variety, lower in restricted food items, and more effective therapeutically. Unfortunately, an undesirable competition between drug and diet therapy exists. Diet therapy is handicapped because it requires a knowledge of a field in which the physician is not trained, more patient cooperation, and more physician time.

We believe that both forms of therapy have a role to play in managing hypertension, and that better results are obtained by the proper use of both. Because diet and other living habit therapy have broader therapeutic effects on hypertension and the diseases that frequently accompany hypertension, diet and living habit therapy should be the primary treatment in the vast majority of cases. Indeed, in our experience, living habit changes alone have proved very effective in the control of high blood pressure. Additional treatment with drugs has been necessary in only a minority of the cases.

Drugs are, of course, necessary in very severe or accelerated hypertension. Hopefully, this volume will give the patient and his physician basic knowledge of optimal living habits to enable them to achieve the best combined therapy.

16
Hyperlipoproteinemia (High Blood Fats)

Hyperlipoproteinemias, diseases associated with abnormally high levels of blood fats, are commonly found in the U.S. adult population. The vast majority of these blood fat disorders are a result of diabetes, obesity, hypothyroidism, nephrosis, and faulty eating or living patterns. A small minority of patients fall in the category of hereditary hyperlipoproteinemias.

Five types of hyperlipoproteinemias have been identified by blood analysis (Table 16–1). The principal therapy for all types is dietary. In all, weight reduction to the optimal level, and marked restriction of fat and cholesterol intake are the major principles treatment. In three of the types, the restriction of carbohydrates is also necessary. Treatment with specific drugs is helpful in some types to supplement dietary therapy.

Blood fats are also known as *lipids* (cholesterol and triglycerides). Our diets for these disorders of lipid metabolism are described on the following pages.

Because two types of this disease (Types I & II) are not carbohydrate sensitive, patients with these disorders may add from 25 to 100 grams of carbohydrate (in the form of fruits and vegetables) to their diets after optimal weight is achieved. The caloric range of the diets is from 580 to 1000 calories. For caloric levels of about 1000 use our Optimal Diets without eggs or margarine. Coffee, tea, cola drinks, and alcohol should be avoided.

higher calorie diet is begun. The maintenance calorie level is established by trial and error. The highest level that will not

The choice of the initial diet depends on body weight in relation to optimal weight. For patients more than 35 pounds over optimal weight, we recommend the 580-calorie diet; for those less than 35 pounds over optimal weight, the initial diet is the 1000-calorie one. When optimal weight is reached, the next

cause an increase in body weight above the optimal, or raise blood fat levels above the lowest level achieved, is the goal of therapy.

TABLE 16-1

CLASSIFICATION OF HYPERLIPOPROTEINEMIAS

Type	Clinical	Cholesterol	Triglycerides
I	Rare. Usually familial and in childhood. Plasma creamy. Due to deficiency of lipoprotein lipase, an enzyme that clears chylomicrons from plasma.	Elevated	Markedly elevated (often 5000 mg%)
II*	Common and occurs at all ages. Familial or secondary to high cholesterol diet, nephrosis, or liver disease. Xanthomas and premature vascular disease present.	Elevated (300–600 mg%)	Normal or mildly elevated
III	Uncommon. Usually familial (recessive trait). Xanthoma and premature vascular disease present.	Elevated (385–800 mg%)	Elevated (385–800 mg%)
IV	Very common. Often associated with diabetes mellitus, hyperuricemia, xanthoma, premature vascular disease. Familial or secondary to other metabolic disorders. Aggravated by excessive carbohydrate or alcohol.	Normal or mildly elevated	Elevated
V	Uncommon. Often secondary to acute metabolic disorders (diabetic acidosis, pancreatitis, hyperuricemia, nephrosis), but may be familial. Aggravated by excessive carbohydrates, or alcohol.	Elevated	Elevated (1000–6000 mg%)

*This type has been further divided into subtypes A and B, but this does not affect the diet treatment.

HYPERLIPOPROTEINEMIA DIET (580 CALORIES)

Basic Diet Plan	Sample Menu

Basic Diet Plan

BREAKFAST
1 fruit unit (list 2)
1/2 carbohydrate unit (list 3)
1/2 cup non-fat milk
beverage
water

MID-MORNING
1 fruit unit (list 2)
water

LUNCH
1 ounce protein (list 4)
list 1 vegetables as desired
1/2 carbohydrate unit (list 3)
1/2 cup non-fat milk
beverage
water

MID-AFTERNOON
1 fruit unit (list 2)
water

DINNER
1 ounce protein (list 4)
list 1 vegetables as desired
1/2 carbohydrate unit (list 3)
1 fruit unit (list 2)
1/2 cup non-fat milk
beverage
water

BEDTIME
1/2 fruit unit (list 2)
1/2 cup non-fat milk

Sample Menu

1/2 small grapefruit
1/2 slice toast
1/2 cup non-fat milk
coffee substitute or water

1 large tangerine

1 ounce cottage cheese
large mixed green salad with vinegar
  dressing
1 cup green beans
1/2 slice bread
1/2 cup non-fat milk
hot or iced tea/lemon

1/2 cup orange juice

1 ounce sliced chicken
1 cup cooked broccoli
large tomato and endive salad/lemon
1/2 slice bread
1/2 cup cinnamon applesauce
1/2 cup non-fat milk
coffee substitute

1/2 cup fresh strawberries
1/2 cup non-fat milk

carbohydrate	91 gm	364 calories 62%
protein	33 gm	132 calories 23%
fat	10 gm	90 calories 15%
cholesterol	<150 mg	
salt	<2.5 gm	

HYPERLIPOPROTEINEMIA DIET (1000 CALORIES)

Basic Diet Plan	Sample Menu
BREAKFAST	
1 fruit unit (list 2)	1/2 small grapefruit
1 carbohydrate unit (list 3)	1 slice toast
1/2 cup non-fat milk	1/2 cup non-fat milk
beverage	coffee substitute
water	
MID-MORNING	
1/2 cup non-fat milk	1/2 cup non-fat milk
water	
LUNCH	
1 ounce protein (list 4)	1 ounce cottage cheese
list 1 vegetables as desired	1 large tomato on shredded lettuce
1/2 vegetable (list 3)	1/2 cup cooked carrots
2 carbohydrate units (list 3)	2 slices bread
1 fruit unit (list 2)	12 fresh grapes
1/2 cup non-fat milk	1/2 cup non-fat milk
beverage	coffee substitute or tea
water	
MID-AFTERNOON	
1/2 cup non-fat milk	1/2 cup non-fat milk
water	
DINNER	
1 ounce protein	1 ounce roast chicken
list 1 vegetables as desired	mixed green salad with vinegar
2 carbohydrate units (list 3)	1/2 cup mashed potato
1 vegetable unit (list 3)	1 slice bread
1 fruit unit (list 2)	1 cup pickled beets
1/2 cup non-fat milk	1/2 cup sliced peaches
water	1/2 cup non-fat milk
BEDTIME	
1/2 cup non-fat milk	1/2 cup non-fat milk
1 fruit unit (list 2)	2 fresh plums

carbohydrate	172 gm	688 calories 69%
protein	54 gm	216 calories 22%
fat	10 gm	90 calories 9%
cholesterol	$<$150 mg	
salt	$<$2.5 gm	

Food Exchange List for All Diets

General Rules

1. Eat only foods listed on this diet, and in amounts indicated. Do not skip meals or feedings. Prepare and eat all food without added fat, sugar, salt, or gravy.

2. Use fresh or frozen meats, fish, vegetables, and fruits.

3. Salt & sugar substitutes may be used with your doctor's approval. Drink at least 1 glass of water before or with each meal.

4. Learn the caloric value of everything you eat.

List 1

Miscellaneous very low calorie foods: 25 calories per serving or less.

Seasoning: cinnamon, garlic, lemon, dry mustard, mint, nutmeg, parsley, pepper, sugarless sweeteners, spices, vanilla, vinegar, low-sodium tomato juice.

Salad Dressing: vinegar, lemon, pepper, parsley, garlic, salt substitute, dry mustard.

Other foods: cranberries, diet soft drinks, decaffeinated coffee, coffee substitute (Postum, Breakfast Cup, Sanocaf, etc.).

Vegetables: asparagus, broccoli, brussels sprouts, cabbage, cauliflower, cucumber, eggplant, lettuce, mushrooms, peppers, radishes, string beans, summer squash, tomatoes, watercress, wax beans, celery. summer squash, tomatoes, watercress, wax beans, celery.;

List 2

Fruit: 50 calories per serving

apple	1 (2" dia.)
applesauce	1/2 cup
apricots	2 medium
banana	1 small
strawberries	1 cup
blueberries	2/3 cup
cantaloupe	1/4 (6" dia.)
cherries	10 large
grapefruit	1/2 small
grapefruit juice	1/2 cup
grapes	12
grape juice	1/4 cup
honeydew	1/8 (7")
mango	1/2 small
orange	1 small
orange juice	1/2 cup

peach	1 medium
pear	1 small
pineapple	1/2 cup
pineapple juice	1/3 cup
plums	2 medium
prune juice	1/4 cup
tangerine	1 large
watermelon	1 cup

List 3

Carbohydrate: 70 calories per serving

bread or tortilla	1 slice
roll	1 (2" dia.)
crackers	4 unsalted
cereals, cooked	1/2 cup
dry	3/4 cup
rice, grits, cooked	1/2 cup
beans, lima, navy	1/2 cup
baked	1/4 cup
spaghetti, noodles, macaroni	1/2 cup
corn, lentils, split peas	1/3 cup
potato, white	1 (2" dia.)
onions	1 cup
peas, green	1 cup
winter squash	1 cup
turnips, beets, rutabagas	1 cup
carrots	1 cup

List 4

Protein: 75 calories per serving

Meat: turkey, chicken, veal, lamb, beef: 1 slice (3" x 2" x 1/8" or 1 ounce) *Fish:* bass, bluefish, catfish, cod, flounder, halibut, rockfish, salmon, sole, tuna (fresh, canned in water, or washed with water: same amount as meat).

Low fat cottage cheese: 1/4 cup (use 1 portion only daily). Non-fat milk, jello: 3/4 cup.

Fish and fowl are most desirable. Eat others only one time per week maximum.

17
Diabetes

The advent of oral hypoglycemics (blood-sugar-lowering agents) has resulted in less emphasis on nutritional therapy in diabetes treatments. For many physicians and patients these agents have become a substitute for dietary therapy. The preference of both physicians and patient for an oral medication rather than a change in lifelong eating habits is readily understandable.

The vast majority of physicians have had no training in nutrition and have not kept abreast of advances in the field. Thus, most physicians must rely on the diabetic diets recommended by various professional organizations. These were devised many years ago, and do not take into account the latest knowledge of nutritional-metabolic disorders, or the newer food products that greatly increase the usefulness of nutritional therapy.

There are several major shortcomings to conventional diabetic diets:

• They focus mainly on carbohydrate restriction and blood sugar control.

• They imitate the average U.S. diet (high in cholesterol, saturated fats, salt and calories), which favors the premature development of atherosclerosis.

• The caloric intake is based on recommendations that are too high for achieving or maintaining optimal weights in the sedentary population of the U.S.

Of the three methods of diabetic therapy, the nutritional is the only one capable of *controlling or preventing* the major diseases associated with diabetes: obesity, atherosclerosis, hypertension, coronary artery disease, kidney failure, and hyperlipoproteinemias. Even in the 20% of diabetics who require insulin, diet is essential for satisfactory control and for minimizing complications.

The status of oral medication that lowers blood sugar is controversial. Some authorities advocate their use in many diabetics who do not need insulin, whereas others believe that any diabetic who is controlled by these drugs can be controlled as well by proper diet therapy.

We believe that, more than ever before, nutritional therapy is the keystone of the treatment of the diabetic patient, whether he be in the prediabetic, latent, or overt stage of the disease. The same holds true whether the patient is insulin dependent or not. We recommend that whenever possible the need for and the dosage of hypoglycemic agent be determined *after* the Optimal Diet for each patient has been established.

We use diet for the fine adjustment and the hypoglycemic agent for the coarse adjustment of blood sugar level. Such an approach requires more meticulous attention to, and more knowledge of, nutrition than the average physician has to offer his diabetic patients. After observing several thousand diabetics, we saw that control was far from below optimal, and that the most frequent cause for this was inadequate diet therapy.

The purpose of this chapter is to help the diabetic and the physician improve the treatment of diabetes through the rational use of diets based on the most recent knowledge of nutrition, diabetes, and new food products, as tested by us in hundreds of diabetic patients.

Our diets are designed to:

● Achieve and maintain optimal weight.

● Achieve maximum acceptability by imitating the optimal diet of the healthy person.

● Control blood fats, blood pressure, heart and kidney function, as well as blood sugar.

● Minimize fluctuations in blood sugar.

● Establish optimal control with minimal caloric intake and minimal dosage of insulin.

Our method of establishing the optimal diabetic diet is as follows:

● Estimate optimal weight (Chapter 1), and calculate the excess weight over optimal.

● Estimate the level of physical activity according to the following three categories: Low (bedridden or confined to home), Moderate (fully active in a sedentary job), High (job requiring above average physical activity and physical activities in addition to job).

● The choice of the initial diet according to these criteria is shown in Table 17–1.

TABLE 17–1

CHOICE OF INITIAL DIET FOR THE DIABETIC

Weight	Activity	Diet
More than 100 lbs. over optimal	low	Obesity Diet 2 or 3
	moderate	Obesity Diet 3
35–100 lbs. over optimal	low	Obesity Diet 2 or 3
	moderate	Obesity Diet 3 or 4
Less than 35 lbs. over optimal	low	Obesity Diet 3 or 4
	moderate or high	Obesity Diet 4
optimal	low	Optimal Diet 2
	moderate	Optimal Diet 3 or 4
	high	Optimal Diet 4 or 5

When the patient achieves optimal weight, he is started on **Optimal Diet 2** (Chapter 10), and this is gradually increased in calories using **Optimal Diets 3–5**. Changes in the diet are made on an individual basis to achieve and maintain optimal weight, as well as optimal levels of blood sugar, blood lipids, blood pressure, and patient satisfaction with the diet.

All of the diets are low in cholesterol, saturated fat, and salt. If edema, hypertension, heart disease, and kidney disease are not present, the salt intake may be increased to up to five grams per day if the patient desires. Use of substitute salt is permitted.

Every effort is made to avoid low blood sugar reactions and glycosuria (sugar spillage in urine) by dietary rather than drug changes. This is achieved by changing the size of the meals that affect the hypoglycemic or hyperglycemic (high blood sugar) episodes; e.g., the meal immediately preceding a hypoglycemic episode is increased, and the meal immediately preceding the hyperglycemic episode is decreased in caloric content without changing the daily caloric intake.

Note that our diabetic diets are identical to the obesity diets at the lower calorie levels and to the optimal or extra-calorie diets at the middle and higher caloric levels. However, the non-

diabetic groups are allowed restricted foods, (eggs, other saturated fat foods, and concentrated carbohydrate foods) more
often: two to four times per week rather than one time per
week for the diabetic.

18
Cancer

Cancer is one of the great concerns of our age, in terms of individual health and national wealth. Twenty-five percent of the U.S. population will develop some form of cancer, and 20% will die of it. Direct patient costs now range between $10,000 and $40,000, and with the progress of medical research these costs can only rise.[64] The best way to reduce incidence of cancer may be to modify our external and internal environment, including nutrition.

What evidence demonstrates that cancer may be preventable? The incidence of certain cancers, such as skin cancer, may be a hundred times as high in one country as another (e.g., U.S.A. compared to India). Typically, the variation between countries of a given cancer, is greater than 100%. This suggests that environmental or noninherited factors are the most probable cause, with nutrition as a major environmental factor. Epidemiological studies by Dr. Ernest Wynder suggest that nutrition may account for as much as 50% of all cancers.[65]

Dr. Wynder lists three ways nutrition can affect cancer:

- Nutrients as carcinogens (promoters of cancer).
- Dietary deficiencies leading to biochemical malfunctions.
- Nutritional excesses that induce metabolic abnormalities.

Epidemiology

Epidemiologists relate the incidence of cancer to different cultures or lifestyles. Their work provides clues to environmental causes of cancer, which can then be followed up by other scientific disciplines. The marked variations between cultures are illustrated by the following statistics.[66]

Cancer	Incidence
Esophagus	Iran 300 times Nigeria
Skin	USA 150 times India
Stomach	Japan 50 times Uganda
Liver	Mozambique 70 times Norway
Rectum	Denmark 50 times Nigeria
Colon	USA 30 times Nigeria & 10 times Japan

These data powerfully suggest prevention is a practical possibility.

There is also considerable evidence that these differences are not racial. Esophageal cancer is very common in East Africa, but is almost unknown in West Africa. San Francisco Japanese, in comparison to Japanese in Japan have:

- 1/4 the gastric cancer (male)
- 3 to 4 times the cancer of the colon (male)
- 3 times the cancer of the breast (female)
- 5 times the cancer of the prostate (male)

Frequently, differences of cancer prevalence in a given locality can be associated with lifestyle factors. For example, those with esophageal cancer in New York City tend to be heavier smokers and drinkers, and consume less milk and green and leafy vegetables.[67]

Sometimes a specific nutritional or metabolic condition can be clearly associated with a very high incidence of a specific cancer. Cancer of the liver, for example, affects 10–30% of Bantu males in Saharal Africa. This exceptionally high rate, which is 500 times that observed in the USA, has been associated with dietary contamination with afltoxin.

In contrast to specific effects from specific nutrients, certain general nutritional factors may be associated with a generalized susceptibility to cancer. For example, actuarial studies have shown a positive correlation between body weight and cancer of all types, but especially of cancers of the intestinal and genitourinary tracts.[68]

The low incidence of all forms of cancer in Seventh Day Adventists suggest nutritional, or perhaps multiple lifestyle influences. The distinctive lifestyle elements of the Seventh Day Adventists are: vegetarianism (50% are lacto-ovo-vegetarian; 80% are at least near vegetarian); nonsmoking; nondrinking;

concern for family life; lower obesity; health education; avoidance of coffee, tea, or spices; 25% less fat and 50% more fiber; and a P/S (polysaturated to saturated fat) ratio twice that of the typical American. Their cancer rate is 50 to 70% of the average USA population. In comparison to the U.S.A. average, Seventh Day Adventists have:

Cancer	Percent of USA Average
Larynx	2%
Esophagus	34%
Bladder	23%
GI Tract	68%
Reproductive	71%
CNS	113%
Leukemia	60%
Kidney	98%

Which lifestyle factors might account for these differences? We have confidence in the association between smoking and several of the above cancers. Statistical analysis has apparently eliminated possible differences due to education or economic level. However, study of 100,000 California Seventh Day Adventists did support the hypothesis that beef, meat, and saturated fat, in general, are related to colon cancer (fiber showed no significant correlation), and that breast cancer seemed to be associated with fried foods.[69]

A factor not considered in these reviews was obesity, though obesity has been shown to be positively correlated with most cancers. Because Seventh Day Adventists have a lower prevalence of obesity, this might partially account for the lower rates. However, the studies of Adventists and of Japanese migrants do point strongly to other lifestyle factors as well. For example, the results of Adventist vegetarian diets are, in addition to less obesity, higher Vitamin C and A, lower exposure to additives, lower intake of protein, total fat, and saturated fats, and higher intake of fiber.

Prevention

It is beginning to appear that certain casual and protective agents can be identified, that have a fairly consistent association with cancer, and these may form the basis for general recommendations affecting our lifestyle, food industry, and legislation.

Fat

High fat intake has been associated with cancer of the colon. Studies using rats (Bandaru, 1976) indicate that the type of fat doesn't matter. These studies suggest that high fat modifies the concentration of bile, as well as the composition of intestinal bacteria. Then, bacterial action on the bile salts may lead to cancer-forming compounds. Fat intake may also influence such body functions as food transit time, which then affects the duration of contact of carcinogens (Phillips, 1975). High fat intake is also associated with cancer of the breast (Modan, 1977).

Cellular Protective Mechanisms

A very interesting area of research is on the effect certain nutrients have in enhancing a natural, protective mechanism of certain body organs. This mechanism, termed the "microsomal mixed-function oxidase system," destroys many chemical carcinogens.[70] This system, found mainly in the liver and kidney, appears to detoxify by modifying the carcinogen, so that it can be metabolized by the body.

A number of vegetables have been found to enhance this activity. Among the most effective are *brussels sprouts, cabbage, turnips, broccoli,* and *cauliflower.* Others mentioned are *spinach, dill,* and *celery.* Oddly, certain insecticides, citrus fruits, and BHA (a food additive), also enhance this system.

Finding protective factors in foods may be one of the most promising avenues of prevention, since attempts to encourage major changes in dietary lifestyle have been disappointing.

Alcohol

Though we do not yet understand the mechanism of action, we do know that heavy drinking is associated with cancer of the oropharynx, esophagus, and liver. Since heavy drinkers are nearly always heavy smokers, it is difficult to isolate the cause.

Artificial Sweeteners

Cyclamates were implicated in cancer of the bladder, and

have been removed from the market. Saccharin has been more recently implicated, based on studies using mice. However, the significance of saccharin use in humans is in dispute. Diabetics, for example, known to be high consumers of saccharin, have not been proven to have a greater risk of cancer.

Nitrites

Nitrites are a common additive in preserving meat and fish products. Amines are widely distributed in foods and drugs. If these two chemicals are synthesized in the body, they may be implicated in esophageal and gastric cancer. Further study is needed, but the prudent individual may wish to reduce intake of meats and increase vegetable protein sources.

Recommendations

That nutrition is of major significance in cancer appears to be well supported by scientific studies. Nevertheless, it is difficult to propose dietary recommendations from the studies reported. To be sure, the lack of cancer in Seventh Day Adventists demonstrates that individuals in our soceity can modify their lifestyle and get substantial reduction in risk—even without a clearly optimal diet. As we get a better understanding of the causes of the various cancers, we can design an even better diet.

Nevertheless, on the basis of present evidence, several general recommendations are in order:

• *Reduce body fat:* Weight reduction has a strong association with reduction of cancer. The evidence associating cancer of the colon with high total fat, and the lack of any evidence incriminating low fat, suggests we should markedly reduce the proportion of fat in our diet. This will also support weight loss.

• *Do not increase Vitamin B:* Failure to demonstrate that increases in the B vitamins give any cancer protection, even at nine times MDR, indicates supplementation of these vitamins is not useful. However, there seems to be some evidence favoring nutrients known to reduce the formation of free radicals, such as Vitamins C, E, D, and selenium. More research appears to be necessary before appropriate dosages (if any) can be recommended.

19
Edema
(Fluid Retention)

There are many diseases in which edema is a chronic or recurring problem. These consist of various stages of heart, kidney, and liver diseases, obesity, hyperproteinemia, anemia, and a number of ill-defined edematous states associated with the menstrual cycle, body position, or hormonal imbalance. Notwithstanding the variety of causes involved, the common factors in the control of the edema are sodium intake and output. Progress has occurred during recent years that makes edema control much easier. More potent diuretics (which increase urine flow) have been developed, and a wide variety of palatable food products of low-sodium content are now available.

Diuretics have enjoyed greater popularity than diets because doctors may prescribe them easily and patients comply with them better. This is unfortunate because diuretics have certain drawbacks, and their therapeutic effects can be largely nullified by improper diet. Furthermore, the long-term use of a diuretic may result in electrolyte deficiency, allergy, or resistance.

We believe that diet therapy should play the key role in the control of chronic or intermittent edema. At best, it eliminates the need for diuretics and their possible undesirable side effects. At the very least, it can reduce the dosage and frequency of diuretics to safer levels.

Whereas formerly it was difficult to design a palatable low-sodium diet suitable for long-term use, this is no longer true. The vast array of commercially available low-sodium foods, as well as salt substitutes, makes it possible to design acceptable meals at all desired levels of sodium suitable for long-term use.

DIET 1 (500 MG NA)

(1200 CALORIE LEVEL)

Eat only the amounts of food listed for each unit. Group A vegetables may be eaten as desired since their sodium level is quite low, and their caloric level is negligible. Prepare all food without salt.

List 1: choose 2 units skim milk
List 2: choose 1 each from Groups A, B, and C
List 3: choose 4 units
List 4: choose 5 units
List 5: choose 5 units
List 6: none
List 7: choose 1 unit

SAMPLE MENU

BREAKFAST
1/2 fresh grapefruit
1/2 cup oatmeal
1/2 cup skim milk
2 teaspoons sugar
1 slice low-sodium toast
coffee or tea
MID-MORNING
1 slice low-sodium toast
2 teaspoons jelly
coffee substitute
LUNCH
main dish salad made with:
2 ounces dietetic tuna, 1 medium tomato, 3 large romaine leaves
4 pieces unsalted melba toast
1 medium fresh peach
1/2 cup skim milk
hot or iced tea
MID-AFTERNOON
1/2 cup skim milk
DINNER
3 ounces broiled beef pattie
1/2 cup steamed rice
1/2 cup cooked green peas
cabbage and green pepper slaw with low-sodium, low calorie dressing
1 small low-sodium roll
1/2 cup fresh fruit cup
coffee substitute
BEDTIME
1 small apple or 1/2 cup unsweetened applesauce
1/2 cup skim milk

No salt is to be used in preparation of food and no salt is to be added at the table.

DIET 2 (500 MG NA)
(1800 CALORIE LEVEL)

Eat only the amounts of food listed for each unit. Group A vegetables may be eaten as desired since their sodium level is quite low, and their caloric level is negligible. Prepare all food without salt. No salt is to be added at the table.

List 1: choose 2 units using skim milk
List 2: choose 1 unit from Groups A and B; 2 units from Group C
List 3: choose 4 units
List 4: choose 7 units
List 5: choose 5 units
List 6: choose 4 units
List 7: choose 2 units

SAMPLE MENU

BREAKFAST
1/2 cup grapefruit juice
1 egg, poached or scrambled
1/2 cup cinnamon applesauce
2 slices low-sodium toast
1 small pat unsalted margarine (1 teaspoon)
coffee substitute
MID-MORNING
1/2 cup milk
5 low-sodium crackers
LUNCH
2 ounces sliced chicken
2 slices low-sodium break with 1 teaspoon unsalted margarine
1 tablespoon cranberry sauce
1/2 cup broccoli
1 cup lettuce salad with lemon
1 cup milk
hot or iced tea with lemon
MID-AFTERNOON
1 fresh tangerine
coffee substitute
DINNER
vegetable stock soup with 1/2 cup cooked dried beans
2 ounces broiled halibut with lemon wedge
1 medium broiled tomato with dill seasoning
1/2 cup cooked green peas
1/2 small baked sweet potato
1 small low-sodium corn muffin
2 teaspoons unsalted margarine
rice and raisin pudding made with 1/2 cup cooked rice, 2 tablespoons
   raisins, 1/2 cup milk
coffee substitute
BEDTIME
1/2 cup diced pineapple
hot tea with lemon

FOOD EXCHANGE LISTS FOR SODIUM-RESTRICTED DIETS

(Compiled by a joint committee of the American Heart Association, the American Dietetic Association, and the U.S. Public Health Service, and modified by the authors to meet criteria set up for restrictions other than sodium.)

List 1: Milk Units

Each unit of whole milk: sodium 120 mg. (7 mg if low-sodium milk is used), calories 170, protein 8 gm, fat 10 gm, carbohydrate 12 gm.

Each unit fresh skim milk or not-fat dry milk: sodium 120 mg (7 mg if low-sodium milk is used), calories 85, protein 8 gm, fat negligible, carbohydrate 12 gm.

whole milk	1 cup
evaporated whole	1/2 cup
non-fat dry	3–4 tablespoons (read label directions)
fresh skim or nonfat	1 cup

Avoid

Commerical foods made with milk, ice cream, sherbet, milk shakes, chocolate milk, malted milk, milk mixes, condensed milk.

Note: Nonfat or fresh skim milk are equal to whole milk in caloric and fat values when 2 fat units are added to each milk unit.

List 2: Vegetables

GROUP A. Fresh, frozen, or dietetic canned only—each unit contains 9 mg. sodium. The carbohydrate, protein, and fat levels are negligible. Each unit is a 1/2-cup serving.

asparagus	lettuce
broccoli	mushrooms
brussels sprouts	okra
cabbage	peppers, red or green
cauliflower	radishes
chicory	squash, summer (yellow or zucchini)
cucumber	tomato juice (low-sodium)
endive	tomatoes
escarole	turnip greens
green beans	wax beans

Avoid

Canned vegetables or vegetable juices except low-sodium dietetic:

beet greens	kale
celery	mustard greens
Swiss chard	sauerkraut
dandelion greens	spinach

Note: Two units of vegetables from Group A may be substituted for one unit from Group B.

GROUP B. Each unit contains 9 mg. sodium, 35 calories, protein 2 gm, carbohydrate 7 gm, fat negligible. Each unit is a 1/2 cup serving.
onions
peas (fresh or low-sodium canned)
rutabaga (yellow turnip)
squash, winter (acorn, butternut, or Hubbard)

Avoid

beets
carrots
frozen peas processed with salt brine
canned vegetables except dietetic

GROUP C. Each unit contains 5 mg sodium, 70 calories, 2 gm protein, 15 gm carbohydrate, fat negligible.
1/2 cup dried beans, lima or navy
1/3 cup cooked fresh lima beans
1/4 cup baked beans, no pork
1/3 cup corn (1/2 small ear)
1/2 cup cooked lentils
2/3 cup parsnips
1/2 cup cooked split green or yellow peas or cowpeas
1 small potato, baked white
1/2 cup mashed potato, white
1/4 cup mashed potato, sweet
1/2 small baked sweet potato

Avoid

frozen lima beans processed with salt
all canned vegetables except dietetic low-sodium
potato chips
processed potatoes with sodium added
Note: One unit from the bread list may be substituted for one unit of Group C vegetable.

List 3: Fruits

Unsweetened, fresh, frozen, canned, or dried—each unit contains 2 mg sodium, 50 calories, 10 gm carbohydrate, both fat and protein are negligible.
apple, 1 small
apple cider or juice 1/3 cup
applesauce 1/2 cup
apricots, dried 4 halves
apricots, fresh 2 medium

apricot nectar 1/4 cup
banana 1/2 small
blackberries 1 cup
blueberries 2/3 cup
cantaloupe 1/4 small
cherries 10 large
cranberries, sweetened 1 tablespoon
dates 2
fig 1 medium
fruit cup 1/2 cup
grapefruit 1/2 small
grapefruit juice 1/2 cup
grapes 12
grape juice 1/4 cup
honeydew 1/8 melon
mango 1/2 small
orange 1 small
orange juice 1/2 cup
papaya 1/3 medium
peach 1 medium
pear 1 small
pineapple 2 slices
pineapple 1/2 cup diced
pineapple juice 1/3 cup
plums 2 medium
prunes 2 medium
prune juice 1/4 cup
raisins 2 tablespoons
rhubarb, sweetened 2 tablespoons
strawberries 1 cup
tangerine 1 large
tangerine juice 1/2 cup
watermelon 1 cup

AVOID

all crystallized or glazed fruit
maraschino cherries
dried fruits with sodium sulfite added
Note: Use as desired: fresh lemons and limes and their juices, unsweetened
cranberries and cranberry juice, unsweetened rhubarb.

List 4: Bread

Low-sodium breads, cereals, and cereal products. Each unit contains
5 mg sodium, 70 calories, 2 gm protein, 15 gm carbohydrate, fat level
negligible.

BREADS AND ROLLS (YEAST) MADE WITHOUT SALT
bread 1 slice
melba toast, unsalted 4 pieces
roll 1 medium
breads (quick) made with sodium-free baking powder or potassium bicarbonate and without salt, or made from low-sodium dietetic mix
biscuit 1 medium
cornbread 1 cube 1-1/2 inch
griddle cakes 2/3 inch
muffin 1 medium

Avoid

Yeastbreads, rolls, or melba toast made with salt or from a commercial mix. All quick breads made with baking powder, baking soda, salt, or made from a commercial mix.

CEREALS, UNSALTED, COOKED
farina 1/2 cup
oatmeal 1/2 cup
rolled wheat 1/2 cup
wheat meal 1/2 cup

Avoid

Quick cooking and enriched cereals which contain a sodium compound—READ LABELS!

CEREALS, DRY
puffed rice 3/4 cup
puffed wheat 3/4 cup
shredded wheat 1 biscuit
cornmeal 2 tablespoons
barley 1-1/2 tablespoons, uncooked
cornstarch 2-1/2 tablespoons
crackers, low-sodium 5 2 in. square
flour 2-1/2 tablespoons
macaroni 1/2 cup cooked
noodles 1/2 cup cooked
popcorn, unsalted 1-1/2 cups
rice, brown or white 1/2 cup cooked
spaghetti 1/2 cup cooked
tapioca 2 tablespoons uncooked
waffle, yeast 8 in. square

Avoid

all dry cereals except those listed
self-rising corn meal

graham crackers or any others except low-sodium
salted popcorn
pretzels
all waffles containing salt, baking powder, baking soda, or egg white
Note: one unit from the vegetable list, Group C, may be substituted for
one bread unit.

List 5: Meat

Meat, fish, poultry, eggs, and low sodium cheese and peanut butter. Each
unit contains 25 mg. sodium, 75 calories, 7 gm protein, 5 gm fat, carbohydrate is negligible.
meat, poultry, fresh, canned low sodium, or frozen
1 unit is 1 ounce cooked
beef
chicken
lamb
liver (1 portion in 2 weeks only)
quail
tongue, fresh
veal
turkey

Avoid

Brains or kidneys, all canned, salted, smoked meats, bacon, bologna,
chipped or corned beef, frankfurters, ham, kosher meats, luncheon meats,
salt pork, sausage, smoked tongue.

FISH OR FISH FILLETS, FRESH ONLY
1 unit is 1 ounce cooked
bass
bluefish
catfish
cod
salmon, canned low-sodium dietetic, 1 ounce
tuna, canned low-sodium dietetic, 1 ounce
flounder
halibut
rockfish
salmon
sole
trout
tuna

Avoid

All frozen fish fillets, canned, salted, or smoked fish, anchovies, caviar,
salted and dried cod, herring, canned salmon (except dietetic), sardines,

regular canned tuna (except dietetic), shellfish: clams, lobster, oysters, scallops, shrimp.
cheese, cottage, unsalted, 1/4 cup
cheese, processed, low-sodium 1 ounce
egg, limit 1 per day
peanut butter, low-sodium, 2 tablespoons

Avoid

All other cheese except low-sodium, all peanut butter and peanut butter products except low-sodium.

List 6: Fats

Each unit contains negligible sodium, 45 calories, 5 gm. fat
avocado 1/3 of 4-in. size
butter, unsalted, 1 teaspoon
cream, heavy, sweet or sour, 1 tablespoon
cream, light, sweet or sour, 2 tablespoons
fat or oil, cooking, unsalted, 1 teaspoon
French dressing, unsalted 1 tablespoon
margarine, unsalted 1 teaspoon
mayonnaise, unsalted 1 teaspoon
nuts, unsalted 6 small

Avoid

all salted butter
bacon and bacon fat
salt pork
olives
all commercial French or other dressing except low-sodium
all salted margarines
all commercial mayonnaise except low-sodium
all salted nuts

Free Choice Items

Each item contains 75 calories and very small amounts of sodium
bread list—1 unit
candy, homemade, salt-free or low-sodium, 75 calories
fat list—2 units
fruit list—2 units
sugar, white or brown—4 teaspoons
syrup, honey, jelly, jam, or marmalade—4 teaspoons
vegetable list, Group C—1 unit

Miscellaneous

fruit juice (but count as fruit unit)

lemonade, using sugar from diet, calcium cyclamate or saccharin
milk (but count as milk unit)
Postum
tea

Avoid
all instant cocoa mixes
prepared beverage mixes, including fruit flavored powders
all fountain beverages
malted milk and other milk drinks
commercial candies
commercially sweetened gelatin desserts
regular baking powder
baking soda (sodium bicarbonate)
pudding mixes
molasses
candy, homemade, salt-free or low-sodium
gelatin, plain, unflavored (use fruit allowance)
leavening agents—cream of tartar, sodium-free baking powder, potassium
   bicarbonate, yeast
rennet dessert powder (not tablets)
tapioca (count as bread unit)

Flavoring Aids

allspice
almond extract
anise seed
basil and bay leaf
bouillon cube, low-sodium
caraway and cardamom seeds
chives
cinnamon and cloves
cumin
curry
dill and fennel seeds
garlic
peppermint flavoring
pimiento
poppy seed
poultry seasoning
rosemary
saccharin
sucaryl (calcium salt only)
saffron
sage
salt substitutes (with doctor's
   permission)
ginger
unsalted horseradish
juniper
lemon extract
mace
maple extract
marjoram and mint
mustard, dry
nutmeg
onion, fresh
orange extract
oregano
paprika
parsley
pepper
savory
sorrel
sugar
tarragon and thyme
turmeric
vanilla extract
vinegar
walnut extract

Avoid

regular bouillon cubes
catsup and chili sauce
celery salt, seed, leaves
garlic and onion salt
salted horseradish
all meat extracts, sauces, and tenderizers
monosodium glutamate
prepared mustard
olives
pickles and pickle relish
salt
soy sauce
Worchestershire sauce

FOOD ALLOWANCES FOR
THE 500 MILLIGRAM SODIUM DIET (display)

Food List	1200 calories units	1800 calories units	Unrestricted calories units
milk	2 skim	2 whole	2 whole
vegetables A	1	1	1 or more
vegetables B	1	1	1 or more
vegetables C	1	1	1 or more
fruit	4	4	2 or more
bread	5	7	4 or more
meat	5	5	5 only
fat	0	4	as desired
free choice	1	2	as desired

Adjustments For Higher or Lower Levels of Sodium

The 500 mg. sodium diet may be adjusted for lower or higher levels of sodium as follows:

For 250 mg substitute low-sodium milk for regular milk.

For 1000 mg substitute 2 slices regular salted bread (400 mg.) and 2 teaspoons regular salted margarine or butter (100 mg.) for 2 slices unsalted bread and 2 teaspoons unsalted margarine or butter, *or* use 1/4-teaspoon salt each day at the table to salt food.

For mild sodium restriction allow ordinary salted bread and margarine or butter and regular milk. Omit the salting of food at the table, salty foods such as potato chips, popcorn and nuts, olives, pickles, relishes, meat sauces, smoked or salted meats.

20
Uremia
(Kidney Failure)

During the last fifteen years there has been renewed interest in the dietary approach to uremia. Despite the success of dialysis and kidney transplants in treating uremia, only a small fraction of uremic patients can be treated by these means because of financial and logistic limitations. There are between 100,000–150,000 uremic patients in the U.S. and 12,000 deaths from uremia per year; less than 5% of the total are treated by dialysis and transplantation. The costs: $10,000 for kidney transplant plus $3,000 per year maintenance costs, $23,000 per year for hemodialysis.

Special low-protein diets have yielded highly promising results. Indeed, the results in small groups of cases compare favorably with those of hemodialysis. These dramatic developments raise the hope that a relatively simple, inexpensive, effective form of treatment is available, either alone, or combined with infrequent dialysis, for the 95% of uremic patients for whom dialysis or transplantation is not available.

Low-Protein Diets

Giordano and Giovannetti (1963–64) introduced the concept of a diet for uremia composed of a minimum amount of essential amino acids (18–20 gm protein) and adequate in calories (from fats and carbohydrates) with careful avoidance of proteins high in nonessential amino acids (grains and vegetables).[71] Low-protein fruits and vegetables are allowed and wheat starch (very low protein) was substituted for wheat flour. The objective of the diet was to provide enough essential amino acids to achieve nitrogen balance and replace protein breakdown. Blood urea was shown to be reutilized for the synthesis of nonessential amino acids, thereby lowering elevated blood urea levels. The adequate caloric level achieved with fats and carbohydrates exerted a protein sparing effect which permits a minimal intake of essential amino acid proteins.

The Giordano-Giovannetti (or G-G) diet was successful in small groups of patients with poor kidney function. Good symptomatic relief and prolongation of useful life were achieved. It was also useful in cases with even less kidney function if combined with occasional dialysis. Unfortunately, this diet has several shortcomings that make it unsuitable for widespread use. Its unpalatability and monotony make it unacceptable to many patients for prolonged use. Furthermore, many patients go into negative nitrogen balance with loss of weight and strength.

Fortunately, others have been able to utilize the principle of the G-G diet to design diets more acceptable to the patient for more prolonged use, and which maintain nitrogen balance. Some workers have reported results equal to those of the original G-G diet with their modified diets.[72] One of these modifications using lactoalbumin in the form of electrodialyzed whey is especially noteworthy.[73] Indeed, it may be considered a landmark in the field because the authors were successful in rehabilitating a man with essentially zero kidney function to a useful life for more than three years by the diet, supplemented with peritoneal dialysis at three- or four-week intervals.

All of the current modifications of the G-G diet, though significant improvements, still remain too complex or limited in variety for routine or widespread prolonged use outside the hospital. Continued efforts to achieve easy to follow, cheaper, more palatable, and less monotonous diets, based on the G-G principles, are clearly needed, both for the vast majority of patients with uremia to whom the diet is the only form of therapy possible, and for those on chronic hemodialysis, in order to reduce the frequency of the dialysis.

On the following pages are a series of diets that we have found effective. They are based on the G-G principles and designed by us to be less complex and more acceptable for longer use than published diets.

Low Protein Diets for Uremia

On the 20-, 30-, and 40-gram protein diets, supplementary

vitamins, iron, and 0.5 grams of Methionine (an essential amino-acid) should be given daily.

Only the 20-gram protein diet uses wheat starch bread. All others use low sodium bread.

All food must be eaten if the diets are to be effective. The diets supply enough protein to minimize the breakdown of body protein. Enough of the essential amino acids are supplied with the exception of Methionine, which should be given as a supplement. Necessary calories can be adjusted up or down by giving or removing foods which contain little or no protein; e.g., fat, jelly, sugar, or syrups.

Uremia Diet 1

(20 gm protein, 179 mg sodium, 1604 mg potassium, total
calories 1732)

This diet is quite restricted, and should only be used in severe
renal insufficiency (creatinine clearance 10 ml/min) when the
patient is hospitalized under close medical supervision. It
derives approximately 14 grams of protein from the complete
protein group. The other 6.25 grams come from fruits, cereal,
and vegetables. Wheat starch, which has a very low protein
content, is used instead of regular flour for making bread. No
salt is used in cooking and no salt is added to food when eaten.
No meat protein is allowed. This diet is intended for short-term
use (1 month or less).

Basic Diet Plan

BREAKFAST
1 fruit (list 4A)
1 egg (list 1A)
1 slice wheat starch bread (list 3)
1 teaspoon unsalted fat (list 6)
hot beverage

MID-MORNING
1 fruit juice (list 4A)

LUNCH
Main Plate:
  2 fruits (list 5A)
  1 fruit (list 5B)
  1 tablespoon unsalted
    mayonnaise (list 6)
  1 slice wheat starch bread (list 3)
  1 teaspoon unsalted fat (list 6)
  beverage

MID-AFTERNOON
1 fruit juice (list 4A)

Sample Menu

1/2 cup apple juice
1 egg
1 slice wheat starch toast
1 teaspoon unsalted margarine
tea or coffee

1/2 cup cranberry juice cocktail

Fruit Salad Plate:
  2 canned pear halves,
  2 canned peach halves,
  4 small apricot halves,
  lettuce leaf,
  1 tablespoon unsalted mayonnaise
1 slice wheat starch bread
1 teaspoon unsalted margarine
hot or iced tea

1/2 cup peach nectar

DINNER

1 cereal (list 3)	1/3 cup cooked noodles
1 vegetable (list 2A)	1 raw tomato salad with
1 tablespoon unsalted	1 tablespoon unsalted mayonnaise
mayonnaise (list 6)	1 slice wheat starch bread
1 slice wheat starch bread (list 3)	1 teaspoon unsalted margarine
1 teaspoon unsalted fat (list 6)	1 large slice canned pineapple
1 fruit (list 5A)	1/2 cup vanilla ice cream
1 ice cream (list 7)	3 ounces milk
3 ounces milk (list 1B)	coffee or tea
beverage	

BEDTIME

1 fruit juice (list 4A)	1/2 cup frozen grape juice

Uremia Diet 2

(30 gm protein, 321 mg sodium, 1593 mg potassium,
total calories 1531)

This diet derives 22 grams of protein from the complete protein group. The remaining 8.3 grams come from fruits, cereals, and vegetables. Regular low-sodium bread is used. No salt is used in cooking and no salt is added to food when eaten. No meat protein is allowed. Ice cream of any flavor (12.5% butterfat type) may be substituted for the protein from the complete protein group (e.g., egg, milk): 1 pint ice cream is equal to 16 grams protein. This diet is intended for limited use; e.g., 1–3 months.

Basic Diet Plan   **Sample Menu**

BREAKFAST

1 fruit (list 4A)	1/2 glass apple juice
1 cereal (list 3)	1/2 cup cooked farina
5 ounces milk (list 1B)	5 ounces milk
2 tablespoons sugar (list 7)	2 tablespoons sugar
beverage	coffee or tea

MID-MORNING

1 fruit juice (list 4A)	1/2 cup cranberry juice cocktail
2 teaspoons sugar (list 7)	2 teaspoons sugar

LUNCH
1 egg (list 1A)	1 poached egg
1/2 bread (list 3) low-sodium	1/2 slice low sodium toast
1 teaspoon unsalted fat (list 6)	1 teaspoon unsalted margarine
1 fruit (list 5A)	2 pear halves
beverage	tea with lemon
1 tablespoon sugar (list 7)	1 teaspoon sugar

MID-AFTERNOON
1 fruit juice (list 4A)	1/2 cup grape juice
1 teaspoon sugar (list 7)	1 teaspoon sugar

DINNER
1 vegetable (list 2C)	baked potato with
1 tablespoon unsalted fat (list 6)	1 tablespoon unsalted margarine
1 vegetable (list 2B)	1/3 cup asparagus
1/2 bread (list 3) low sodium	1/2 slice low-sodium bread
1 teaspoon unsalted fat (list 6)	1 teaspoon unsalted margarine
1 ice cream (list 7)	1/2 cup ice cream
6 ounces milk (list 1B)	6 ounces milk
beverage	tea or Sanka
1 tablespoon sugar (list 7)	1 tablespoon sugar

BEDTIME
1 fruit juice	1/2 cup cranberry juice
2 teaspoons sugar (list 7)	2 teaspoons sugar

Uremia Diet 3

(30 gm protein, 228 mg sodium, 1414 mg potassium,
total calories 1523)

This diet derives 22.0 grams of protein from the complete protein group. The remaining 8.2 grams come from fruits, cereals, and vegetables. Regular low-sodium bread is used. No salt is used in cooking and no salt is added to food when eaten. This diet is similar to Diet 2 except that meat protein is permitted. Meat (including fowl or fish) should be restricted to 2 times per week at first, and gradually increased to 3 or 4 times per week provided no increase in the uremia occurs. Ice cream of any flavor (12.5% butterfat type) may be substituted for the protein from the complete protein group (e.g., egg, milk): 1 pint ice cream is equal to 16 grams protein. This diet is suitable for long term use in patients with marked uremia (creatinine clearance < 10 ml/min).

Basic Diet Plan	Sample Menu
BREAKFAST	
1 fruit juice (list 4A)	1/2 glass apple juice
1 cereal (list 3)	1/2 cup cooked farina
4 ounces whole milk (list 1B)	4 ounces whole milk
2 tablespoons sugar (list 7)	2 tablespoons sugar
hot beverage	coffee or tea
MID-MORNING	
1 fruit juice (list 4A)	1/2 cup cranberry juice
1 teaspoon sugar (list 7)	1 teaspoon sugar
LUNCH	
1 ounce poultry (list 1B)	1 ounce cooked turkey
1 vegetable (list 2B)	1/2 cup green beans
1 vegetable (list 2A)	1 medium tomato on lettuce leaf
1 tablespoon unsalted oil (list 6)	1 tablespoon oil dressing
1/2 slice low sodium bread (list 3)	1/2 slice low sodium bread
1 teaspoon unsalted fat (list 6)	1 teaspoon unsalted margarine
1 tablespoon jelly (list 7)	1 tablespoon jelly
1 fruit (list 5A)	2 canned pear halves
hot beverage	tea with lemon
1 tablespoon sugar (list 7)	1 tablespoon sugar
MID-AFTERNOON	
1 fruit juice (list 4A)	1/2 cup canned grape juice
DINNER	
1 egg (list 1A)	1 poached egg
1 vegetable (list 2B)	1/3 cup cooked asparagus
1/2 slice low sodium bread (list 3)	1/2 slice low sodium bread
1 teaspoon unsalted fat (list 6)	1 teaspoon unsalted margarine
1 tablespoon jelly (list 7)	1 tablespoon jelly
1/2 cup ice cream (list 7)	1/2 cup vanilla ice cream
hot beverage	hot tea or Sanka
1 tablespoon sugar (list 7)	1 tablespoon sugar
BEDTIME	
1 fruit juice (list 4A)	1/2 cup cranberry juice
1 teaspoon sugar (list 7)	1 teaspoon sugar

Uremia Diet 4

(40 gms protein, 329 mgs sodium, 1849 mgs potassium,
total calories 1619)

This diet derives 27 grams of protein from the complete protein group. The remaining 13.4 grams come from fruits, cereals, and vegetables. Regular low sodium bread is used. No salt is used in cooking and no salt is added to food when eaten. Meat is allowed up to 4–6 times per week provided no increase in the uremia occurs. Ice cream of any flavor (12.5% butterfat type) may be substituted for the protein from the complete protein group (e.g., egg, milk): 1 pint ice cream is equal to 16 grams protein. This diet is designed for lifelong use by the uremic patient of moderate to marked severity (creatinine clearance 8–20 ml/min). If the uremia worsens, Diet 3 should be used.

Basic Diet Plan

BREAKFAST
1 fruit (list 4B)
1 cereal (list 3)
1 teaspoon sugar (list 7)
1 bread (list 3) low sodium
1 teaspoon unsalted fat (list 6)
4 ounces milk (list 1B)
hot beverage

MID-MORNING
1 fruit juice (list 4A)

LUNCH
1 egg (list 1A)
1 vegetable (list 2A)
1 vegetable (list 2B)
1 teaspoon unsalted oil (list 6)
1/2 bread (list 3) low sodium
1 teaspoon unsalted fat (list 6)
1 fruit (list 5B)
beverage

MID-AFTERNOON
1 fruit (list 5A)

Sample Menu

1/2 cup apricot nectar
1/2 cup oatmeal
1 teaspoon sugar
1 slice low sodium toast
1 teaspoon unsalted margarine
4 ounces milk
coffee or tea

1/2 cup cranberry juice cocktail

1 scrambled egg
1 medium broiled tomato
1/2 cup shredded cabbage slaw with
    1 teaspoon oil and vinegar dressing
1/2 slice low sodium bread
1 teaspoon unsalted margarine
3 canned plums
tea with lemon

1/2 cup applesauce

DINNER
1 ounce poultry (list 1B)
1 starch (list 3)
1 vegetable (list 2B)
1 fruit (list 5A)
1 tablespoon unsalted
  mayonnaise (list 6)
1/2 bread (list 3) low sodium
1 teaspoon unsalted fat (list 6)
3 ounces ice cream (list 7)
4 ounces milk (list 1B)
beverage

1 ounce roast chicken
1/2 cup noodles
1/2 cup green beans
1 medium chopped apple on lettuce
  leaf
1 tablespoon unsalted mayonnaise
1/2 slice low sodium bread
1 teaspoon unsalted margarine
3 ounces vanilla ice cream
4 ounces milk
tea or Sanka

BEDTIME
1 fruit (list 4A)

1/2 cup frozen grape juice

Uremia Diet 5

(51 gm protein, 533 mg sodium, 3551 mg potassium,
total calories 1807)

This diet derives 35.0 grams of protein from the complete
protein group. The remaining 15.6 grams come from fruits,
cereals, and vegetables. Regular low sodium bread is used. No
salt is used in cooking and no salt is added to food when eaten.
Meat protein is allowed 5–7 times per week. Ice cream of any
flavor (12.5% butterfat type) may be substituted for the protein
from the complete protein group (e.g., egg, milk): 1 pint ice
cream is equal to 16 grams protein. This diet is designed for
lifelong use in patients with mild to moderate degrees of uremia
(creatinine clearance 20–60 ml/min). If the uremia worsens,
change to Diet 4.

Basic Diet Plan

Sample Menu

BREAKFAST
1 fruit (list 4B)
1 bread (list 3)
1 teaspoon unsalted fat (list 6)
1 cereal (list 3)
1 tablespoon sugar (list 7)
6 ounces milk (list 1B)
beverage

1/2 cup orange juice
1 slice toasted low sodium bread
1 teaspoon unsalted margarine
1/2 cup oatmeal
1 tablespoon sugar
6 ounces milk
tea or coffee

MID-MORNING
1 fruit juice (list 4A)

1/2 cup apple juice

LUNCH
1 egg (list 1A)	1 egg omelet
2 vegetables (list 2A)	2 broiled tomato halves
1 vegetable (list 2C)	1 small baked potato
2 fruits (list 5A & list 5B)	salad:
1 tablespoon unsalted	1 stalk celery,
mayonnaise (list 6)	1/2 cup mixed grapefruit & orange
1/2 bread (list 3)	sections,
1 teaspoon unsalted fat (list 6)	1/2 small apple
6 ounces milk (list 1B)	1 tablespoon unsalted mayonnaise
	1/2 slice low sodium bread
	1 teaspoon unsalted margarine
	6 ounces milk

MID-AFTERNOON
1 fruit juice (list 4A)	1/2 cup cranberry cocktail

DINNER
1 ounce fish (list 1B)	1 ounce broiled fish
1 vegetable (list 2B)	1/2 cup cooked carrots
1 vegetable (list 2C)	1/2 cup mashed potato
1 bread (list 3)	1 slice low sodium bread
1 teaspoon unsalted fat (list 6)	1 teaspoon unsalted margarine
1 ice cream (list 7)	1/2 cup vanilla ice cream
5 ounces milk (list 1B)	5 ounces milk
beverage	tea or coffee substitute

BEDTIME
1 fruit juice (list 4A)	1/2 cup grape juice

Food Exchange Lists for Uremia Diets

1. Meat, fish, egg, and milk (7 gm protein). Choose 2 servings to be divided during the day.

A. egg	1 large
B. beef, medium fat	1 oz.
lamb, medium fat	1 oz.
fresh pork	1 oz.
veal	1 oz.
chicken or turkey	1 oz.
fish, without salt	1 oz.
milk, whole	1 oz.

Avoid: All salted, cured, or smoked meats, fish, and poultry as ham, bacon, corned beef, dried beef, frankfurters, and other sausages, luncheon meats, sardines, and herring. All canned meats, poultry, and fish unless labeled "low sodium." All pre-cooked shell fish as shrimp, lobster, crab. All fresh shell fish except shrimp. All frozen prepared TV dinners.

2. *Vegetables.* Use a variety of vegetables so that you may stay within the limits of the prescribed amounts of sodium and potassium.

A. *Raw:* approximately 1 gm protein per serving in quantity listed.

avocado	1/4 pear
cabbage, raw, shredded	1/2 cup
carrots, raw	2 small or 1 large
celery, raw (diced)	3/4 cup
cucumbers, raw, 1/8" thick	8 slices
lettuce, iceberg, shredded	1 cup
onions, bulb, raw	size of egg
onions, green, 5" long	10
peppers, bell, green	1 shell
tomatoes	1 medium

B. *Cooked:* approximately 1 gm protein per serving in quantity listed.

The vegetables used may be fresh or frozen. If canned vegetables are used, they should be the diet pack kind, canned without salt. When cooking fresh or frozen vegetables, cover them with water, then discard the water after cooking them.

asparagus, cut pieces	1/3 cup
green beans, fresh	1/2 cup
green beans, canned	1/2 cup
wax beans, fresh	1/2 cup
wax beans, canned	1/2 cup
beets, fresh	1/2 cup
beets, canned	1/2 cup
cabbage, shredded	1/2 cup
carrots, fresh	3/4 cup
celery, bleached	3/4 cup
eggplant, 3/4" slice	2 slices
mushrooms, fresh	5 small
okra, fresh	1/2 cup
onions	1/2 cup
parsnips, fresh	1/2 cup
rutabaga, fresh	1/2 cup
squash, zucchini, crookneck	1/2 cup
squash, banana, Hubbard, acorn, boiled	1/2 cup

tomatoes, canned	1/2 cup
tomatoes, puree, low sodium	3 tbsp.
turnips, fresh	3/4 cup

C. *Cooked:* Approximately 2 gm. protein per serving in quantity listed.

The vegetables included in this list are higher in protein and should be used less frequently. They may be used fresh or frozen. If canned vegetables are used, they should be the diet pack kind, canned without salt. When cooking the vegetables, cover them with water and discard the water after they are cooked.

broccoli	1 small stalk
brussels sprouts	4 medium
corn	1/2 ear or 1/3 cup
mustard greens	1/2 cup
peas, green canned	1/4 cup
potato, white	1 sm. or 1/2 cup
potato, sweet	1 sm. or 1/2 cup
spinach	1/3 cup

Avoid: All canned vegetables unless labeled "packed without salt." All canned vegetable juices except tomato juice labeled "no salt added." Frozen peas, lima beans, and mixed vegetables. Use fresh celery, carrots, beets, beet greens, and other greens in very small servings. Canned sweet and white potatoes, commercial prepared potatoes, potato chips, frozen potato pancakes, etc.

3. *Bread and Cereal.* Approximately 2 gm. protein per serving in quantity listed.

bread, white, low sodium	1 slice
puffed rice	1 cup
puffed wheat	1 cup
shredded wheat	1 biscuit
sugar-coated cereal	1 cup
rice, cooked	1/2 cup
oatmeal, cooked	1/2 cup
cream of wheat	1/2 cup
spaghetti, cooked	1/3 cup
macaroni, cooked	1/3 cup
noodles, cooked	1/3 cup
wheat starch bread (0.2 gm. protein)	1 slice

---

*Persons on the 20 gm. protein diet should use the wheat starch bread and wheat starch products instead of bread made from wheat flour.

Avoid: All commercial baked breads except those labeled "low sodium," rolls, biscuits, muffins, cornbread, wheat tortillas. All commercial bread mixes, biscuit mixes, muffin mixes, cornbread mixes, roll mixes, pancake mixes, etc. All commercial prepared dough ready to bake. All crackers. All quick cooking cereals not listed in the Bread and Cereal list. Popcorn.

4. *Fruit Juices*

A. Each serving as listed contains approximately 0.2 gm protein.

apple juice, canned	1/2 cup
cranberry juice cocktail	1/2 cup
grape juice, canned or bottled	1/2 cup
grape juice, frozen	1/2 cup
peach nectar, canned	1/2 cup
pineapple and grapefruit drink	1/2 cup
pineapple and orange drink	1/2 cup

B. Each serving as listed contains approximately 0.4 gm protein.

apricot nectar, canned	1/2 cup
lemon juice, fresh	1/2 cup
lime juice, fresh	1/2 cup
pear nectar, canned	1/2 cup
pineapple juice, canned	1/2 cup
orange juice, fresh or canned	1/2 cup
(1/2 cup contains 0.84 gm. protein)	
grapefruit juice, fresh or canned	1/2 cup
(1/2 cup contains 0.6 gm protein)	

5. *Fruits*

A. Each serving as listed contains approximately 0.3 gm. protein.

apples, raw (2 3/4" diameter)	1 medium
applesauce, canned	1/2 cup
cranberries, raw	1 cup
grapes, Thompson, seedless	10–12 medium
nectarine, raw	1 medium
peaches, canned heavy syrup	2 medium (halves)
pear, canned heavy syrup	1/2 cup
pineapple, raw, cubed	1 large slice
pineapple, canned heavy syrup	1/4 cup
raspberries, sweet frozen	1/4 cup
strawberries, frozen	

B. Each serving as listed contains approximately 0.6 gm protein.

apricots, raw	1 large
apricots, canned heavy syrup	4 medium (halves)
bananas	1/2 small
blackberries, raw	1/3 cup
blackberries, canned heavy syrup	1/3 cup
blueberries	1/2 cup
blueberries, frozen unsweetened	1/2 cup
blueberries, canned heavy syrup	1/2 cup
boysenberries, raw	1/3 cup
cantaloupe, raw (5″ diameter)	1/4
cherries, sweet raw	8
cherries, sweet canned	1/3 cup
cherries, red sour, unsweetened	1/3 cup
figs, raw	1 large
figs, canned heavy syrup	1/2 cup
fruit cocktail, canned	1/2 cup
grapefruit, raw (4 1/2″ diam.)	1/2 medium
grapefruit, canned	1/2 cup
oranges, raw (2 1/2″ diameter)	1 small
papaya	1/3 medium
peaches, raw	1 medium
pear, raw	1/2 pear
plums, raw (2″ diameter)	1 plum
plums, purple canned	3 plums
prunes, dried	3 large
raisins, dried	2 tbsp.
raspberries, red raw	1/2 cup
rhubarb, raw cubed	1 cup
rhubarb, frozen sweetened	1/2 cup
strawberries, raw	10 medium
tangerines, raw	1 medium
watermelon, raw, cubed	1/2 cup

Use dried fruits in very small portions.

6. *Fats and Oils*

saltfree butter or margarine
salted butter or margarine
vegetable oil
mayonnaise, saltfree
mayonnaise, salted
sour cream
mocha mix
heavy cream

Avoid: Salted margarine and butter. Bacon fat. All commercial mayonnaises and salted dressings except those labeled "low sodium."

7. *Sweets and Desserts*

honey
jam
jellies
maple syrup
sugar, white
sugar, light brown
vanilla ice cream
sherbet
Hershey chocolate syrup
Danish dessert
cranberry jelly

Avoid: All commercial pies, pastries, cakes, and cookies. All commercial pudding mixes. All Jello type desserts except Danish dessert made with water. All commercial cake, cookie, and pastry mixes. Buttermilk, instant cocoa mixes, soda water, softened water. Baking powder, baking soda, alkalizers, salt, salt substitutes, seasoned salts, seasoned salt substitute, Accent. All condiments as catsup, chili sauce, Worchestershire sauce, steak sauces, prepared mustard except those labeled "low sodium." All pickles, olives. No nuts allowed except when calculated into a recipe. Peanut butter. All canned soups. Bouillon cubes. Low sodium bouillon cubes.

Recipes for Uremic Diets

Yeast-Leavened Rolls or Bread

12 gm sucrose
3 gm sodium chloride
125 gm water (100°F)
9 gm compressed yeast
5 gm salt free margarine
5 gm hydrogenated unsalted fat
0.5 gm glyceryl monosterate
2 drops pure glycerol
150 gm wheat starch

Place sucrose and sodium chloride in mixing bowl and add water. Dissolve yeast in solution. Melt margarine and vegetable fat together. Add glyceryl monostearate to hot fat mixture and stir until dissolved. Add glycerol. Add this mixture to yeast mixture. Add wheat starch, one half at a time, stirring gently on low speed of mixer until starch is well moistened. Mix 5 to 7 minutes with mixer. Scrape sides with spatula once during mixing, but do not scrape beater blades. Remove from mixer and cover bowl with a damp cloth. Allow to ferment 30 minutes at 82° F. At end of 30 minutes, stir mixture by hand until batter turns to the semifluid state it was in before fermentation.

To make rolls, divide batter into 6 aluminum baking muffin cups, well greased with vegetable fat. Brush top of each with melted salt free margarine. If making loaves, pour mixture into a heavy greased aluminum pan (7-1/2 x 3-1/2 x 2-1/2 inches). Brush top with melted salt free margarine.

Cover with damp cloth and let rise 45 minutes at 82° F.

Bake rolls at 400° F. for 20 minutes, place under broiler for 2 minutes to brown tops. Bake loaves at 550° F. for 5 minutes, then at 400° F. for 35 minutes. Place under broiler 2 minutes to brown top. Remove from oven and cool on wire rack.

Composition:
1 loaf after baking—243 gm
6 rolls after baking—228 gm
Each batch of dough contains:
   660 calories
   143 gm carbohydrate
   1.7 gm protein
   9 gm fat

Wheat Starch Cookies

3/4 cup salt free margarine
1 3/4 cup wheatstarch
3 tablespoons granulated sugar
1/2 cup light corn syrup
1 teaspoon vanilla
1/2 teaspoon baking powder

Soften margarine in mixing bowl. Cream together with sugar and corn syrup. Add vanilla. Gradually add wheatstarch, blending well after each addition. Press dough into a roll between waxed paper. Chill. Slice and place on greased baking sheet.

Bake for 15 to 20 minutes in a 325° oven until brown. Makes 4 dozen small cookies.

Each cookie contains 37 calories.

Minute trace sodium

1 mg. potassium

Minute trace protein

Part Five:
Overcoming Stress

21
Defining Stress

"Stress" means different things to different people. Everyone has it and talks about it, but few have a clear understanding of it. "Stressors" (stressful events) are any changes in the world around us. Any excitement is a stress from the physiologist's point of view. Examples of stressors are: temperature changes, hunger, physical activity, sounds, good news, bad news, etc. "Stress" is our body's state of arousal in response to these stressors. It is the sum total of reactions that take place in the body and mind in response to a stressor.

Stress is an inevitable part of living; it cannot be avoided. Only death results in the complete absence of stress. In many ways stress is a desirable and positive force in our lives, to be sought after and enjoyed. Hans Selye, a scientist who has devoted his life to the study of stress, calls it "the spice of life." Successful activity provides exhilaration and maintains youthful feeling and strength. Inactivity results in deterioration of mind, body and spirit. Stress is the stimulus and challenge for successful activity.

In other ways stress can be a negative, tiring, destructive force. In everyday conversation stress is used to mean excessive strain or distress. Distress often results from prolonged stress or frustration. Daniel Goleman, a psychologist doing research on the effects of meditation, says that those who are able to handle stress effectively respond initially to the stressor with a high state of arousal.[74] But as soon as the stressful event is over they rapidly recover and relax. In contrast, the chronically anxious person is equally aroused, but remains so long after the stressful event, thus dissipating his energy.

Each of us has an optimal level of stress, sufficient to stimulate and challenge us to work and to enjoy life to our optimal level, but not enough to overtax us and endanger our health.

According to Selye, each of us has a fixed amount of vitality (adaptive energy) determined by heredity, which may be spent to satisfy our inborn urge for self-expression and survival.

Physiological Reactions to Stress

We experience the stress reaction as a racing heart, quickened breathing, sweating, dry mouth, a sinking sensation in the stomach, faintness, nausea, generalized muscle tension, nervousness, anxiety, etc. Many of these symptoms are due to excess adrenalin, a hormone secreted (released) by the adrenal gland and certain nerve endings in response to stressful situations. It is important to understand, that though the stress reaction is similar in everyone, there is considerable variation between individuals in their susceptibility to stressful circumstances and in the degree of body-mind response to a given stressor. This is especially true of psychological stressors. Some persons have literally died of fright whereas others in a similar situation react with cool detachment, perhaps even enjoying the thrill of a frightening situation. These differences are partly genetic (hereditary) and partly learned (conditioned). We are born with different sensitivities and capacities, yet we have virtually an unlimited potential to learn and to adapt.

Psychological Links

The stress reaction is a primitive adaptive system designed to deal constructively with the changing demands of the environment. The system prepares the body to deal with emergencies. It has been called the "fight or flight" mechanism and is essential for survival in physically dangerous situations. Our difficulties arise when fighting or running away are inappropriate responses to the problem at hand and where we have not developed effective methods of discharging the accumulated tensions.

Thomas Holmes, a psychiatrist, noted that people tended to get sick "when clusters of major events took place in their lives," such as death of a spouse, divorce, marriage, or retirement. Dr. Holmes studied the case histories of over 5000 patients. There was a clumping of life changes just before the onset of major illness. It didn't matter whether these changes were desirable or undesirable—all events accumulated stress.[75]

Inhibition and Stress

Why are humans susceptible to stressful events? Stressors are common to man and animals, but animals in their natural habitat react very differently from man. The difference is how man handles the stress situation. Under threat, a tiger crouches and springs, a snake coils and strikes, the rabbit tenses then flees to the bushes. In each, we observe an accumulation of excitement followed by its discharge through action appropriate to the animal.

Modern man is taught to control his excitement, but is inhibited from discharging this energy through action. If the excitement-energy is not expended, the body tends to remain in a state of alarm, characterized by taut muscles and altered body chemistry. Frustrated from external outlet, the body will continue to seek some outlet, some means of discharge of pent-up energy. A common course is to direct the energy inward, especially toward organ systems susceptible to emotional states: the heart, the gut, and the musculo-skeletal system. This increases the likelihood of disease in these organs.

Outlets for Stress

This is not to say that we have no choice in this matter. We are vulnerable, but we can choose lifestyles and practices that provide healthy outlets for discharge of accumulated tension. Any form of action discharges energy. However, certain actions have a more logical relationship to the source of excitement. Also, the kind of excitement we develop depends on our unique reaction to the stressful event. Two sales people might react quite differently to an unreasonable customer, one with humor and curiosity, another with inner wrath. Their physiological reactions to the same stressor are correspondingly different.

One person may find healthy discharge of pent-up anger through competitive sports. Another, who works all day at a desk and feels frustrated by inactivity, may find that walking, jogging, dancing, or T'ai Chi provides a refreshing relief of tension. A worker on a physically active, but boring, production line may discover balancing outlets in a game of chess or some intellectually challenging hobby. It is important to realize there are no ideal recreational activities universally effective for everyone.

What is the relationship between stress and disease? Some medical authorities speak of "stress diseases" as if certain diseases are clearly linked to stress. Other authorities believe that stress may be a factor in every disease, either beneficial to the progress of the disease or detrimental. It may well be that both concepts are valid.

22
Stress-Busters

"A house divided against itself cannot stand," said Abraham Lincoln. Our tensions and anxieties signify a similar war of internal conflict. We have all experienced this wasted energy of tension. We may come home from a stress-ridden workday, utterly exhausted, "all bottled up." Yet, if we take a walk, or play a set of tennis or engage in some other leisure activity our energy may be restored. Accordingly, most of us will benefit by learning some specific methods to release tensions and regenerate our energy.

We experience stress or tension mainly as a feeling, yet if we examine our overall body reactions we will become aware that our muscles are also tense. Tension is a mind-body event, and this is true with all emotions. This suggests that we might relieve our tensions either by dealing with our emotional conflicts or by relaxing our muscles. The approaches to the management of tension that we offer in this chapter are based on this mind-body relationship.

Over the last few decades the public has been exposed to a wide variety of solutions to our tensions: Yoga, psychoanalysis, sensory awareness, tranquilizers, LSD, encounter groups, T-Groups, etc., and more recently, techniques such as T'ai Chi Ch'uan and bioenergetic analysis.

Which is the optimal path for you? Some approaches require years of discipline, frequently a teacher or guru, and often considerable expense. We cannot describe all of these alternatives, nor can we prescribe a single optimal path that suits everyone. Instead, our aim will be to describe a few of the tension-management techniques which appear to be standing the test of time and have a growing following.

Physical Exercise

Exercise deserves special attention as a method for the management of tension and individual growth for a number of reasons. Foremost, perhaps, is its practicality. Most forms of exercise are inexpensive; opportunities for practice are as near as the floor or outside the closest door, and reasonable proficiency can be acquired in a relatively short time. One usually experiences some of the benefits immediately through the sense of relaxation following vigorous physical effort, and the regular practice of exercise is almost universally recommended by authorities. Dr. Paul Dudley White emphasized: "Muscular fatigue, if not excessive, is the best sedative known to man—the best antidote for nervous strain. Sleep is favored and a delicious tranquility results." Many who do endurance activities regularly report a feeling of euphoria, a sense of being "all together."

One of the stresses of modern life, with its excessive noise, crowding, and dissatisfying jobs is pent-up aggression. Physical exercise is a constructive way to vent these feelings. Dr. Kenneth Cooper has over 1000 executives in his jogging program in Dallas, Texas. The primary benefits they report are emotional repose and untroubled sleep.

Dance

In analyzing the therapeutic effect of dance, Alexander Lowen, a psychiatrist, said, "The feeling which underlies the dance is joy." In dancing, one may express one's individuality and one's culture. It is both an individual and a social occasion. In the relief of tension it shares with physical exercise certain physiological benefits, but there are additional possibilities.

Movement and rhythm are fundamental to life. "To live is to move," writes Lowen. "The person who lives pleasurably moves rhythmically, effortlessly, gracefully." Breathing is rhythmic; peristalsis in the gut is rhythmic, our heart beats rhythmically, and there is growing evidence that we are governed quite considerably by various biorhythms within the day and over more extended periods. The unhealthy state is lack of movement and rigidity. Lowen suggests that muscle regidity is the "mechanism of repression," and that neurosis, such as chronic anxiety or

depression, signifies a chronic disturbance of the natural
mobility of the individual.

Breathing Therapy

Breath is life; so it should be of no surprise that our manner
of breathing effects and is affected by every aspect of ourself.
"One must breathe to live," writes Lowen, "and the better one
breathes, the more alive one is." To be wholly alive is to breathe
deeply, to move freely, and to feel fully.

Many people are poor breathers. They tend to breathe with
their chest. This form of breathing tenses the abdominal and
diaphragmatic muscles, which tends to be experienced as emotional tension and anxiety.

The great teachers of India describe four levels of breathing:

1. Chest (mid breathing). In chest breathing the abdominal
muscles remain taut, resisting the downward contraction of the
diaphragm. The lungs are allowed to expand mainly by enlarg-
ing the rib cage, where the ribs expand. Try this now, so that
you can experience it clearly. Tighten your abdominal muscles
and slowly inhale as deeply as you can; then hold it for a
moment. Note the extreme tension and resistance in the abdominal area. Try to sense the stretching and enlargement of the rib
cage, and the inner feelings due to your inability to inhale
completely.

2. Abdominal (slow breathing). In abdominal breathing the
abdominal muscles are relaxed, allowing a relatively full downward movement of the diaphragm. However, the muscles of the
rib cage are tense. To experience this state, hold your upper
arms tight against the side of your ribs to help confine your
intercostal muscles; then inhale, allowing your abdomen to pro-
trude fully foreward. Note your feelings again, as with chest
breathing.

3. Apical (high breathing). In apical breathing both the
abdominal and rib cage muscles are tense. Inhalation is provided mainly through raising the shoulders, which allows only
the apex (upper lobes) of the lungs to fill with air. This is the
area of the lungs that are least supplied with blood capillaries,
thus aggravating the problem. When you try this style, you will
experience the most inadequate breathing.

4. Complete Breath. The "complete breath" eliminates all the limiting features of the other three forms. Your entire respiratory apparatus is used. Before trying it, sit down and breathe in your accustomed manner. Become as aware as you can of your breathing patterns. Are they rhythmical, or irregular? Do they feel easy and pleasurable, or forced and unnatural?

To experience the complete breath try the following exercise:

(1) Sit or stand erect. Breathe through your nostrils, first filling the lower part of your lungs by relaxing your abdomen.

(2) As step 1 progresses, allow your rib cage to expand upward and outward (feel it enlarge).

(3) Toward the end of step 2, allow your shoulder to rise slightly, filling the upper lobes of your lungs (you may feel the muscles above your clavicle contract gently). Do these three steps slowly to the count of six heart beats.

(4) Hold at maximum inhalation for three counts.

(5) Exhale slowly (for the count of 6).

(6) Hold at maximum exhalation for the count of three. Repeat the entire six steps seven times.

There are two general approaches to improving breathing. One is to repeat the above process two or three times daily. Central to this approach is that daily discipline eventually leads to spontaneity, effort to effortlessness. The second approach is to sit in a natural manner, and concentrate on your act of breathing, observing all inner movements and emotional reactions. You merely "let go." Allow your breathing to find its own natural pattern. Do not attempt to control the pattern. The central principle is to allow the automatic self-restorative powers to work.

Progressive Relaxation Exercise (PRE)

This technique was originated in 1934 by Edmund Jacobsen of Harvard University, as an immediate means of dealing with stressful situations and of developing a more relaxed style in everyday living.[77]

Jacobsen believed that emotional tension was associated with contractions of muscle fibers, that the anxiety could be removed by eliminating the muscle contractions. He noted that by tensing and relaxing muscle groups systematically, and by "attending to" the resulting sensations, the individual can virtually eliminate muscle contractions and experience deep relaxation. The system is not difficult to learn, and one immediately experiences the benefits of a more deeply relaxed state.

Aikido

Physical exercises and sports focus almost exclusively on the body. After developing a basic level of conditioning many people feel the need for a more expanded approach, one which offers greater flexibility, grace, expressiveness, and perhaps skills in self-defense. Aikido is designed to do this.

Aikido is a more recent development of a long line of Oriental martial arts, such as Judo, Karate, and T'ai Chi Ch'uan. A secret art of self-defense originally known only to the nobility of Japan, Aikido has been available to the public since World War II. A number of centers (Federations) have developed recently in the United States.

In most martial arts the training is aimed at learning to defeat the enemy. In Aikido the aim is to conquer oneself. To accomplish this one trains for obedience to the laws of nature, so that one who attacks you, attacks nature itself. There is no strain in the execution of Aikido. One lets the opponent "go where he wants to go, bend in the direction he wants to bend as you lead him, and lets him fall where he wants to fall."

Aikido is not merely an art of self-defense, but is interwoven with philosophy, psychology, and art. Proponents believe it is foremost a training of the mind, and results in overall improvement in health and self-confidence.

Sleep

Although we do not know for certain the function of sleep, we are all well aware that deprivation of sleep has a number of undesirable effects. After prolonged wakefulness we experience a mental sluggishness and frequently irritability. Individuals forced to remain awake in experiments have even developed psychotic symptoms, states of unreality. We can assume from this that sleep restores normal balance in our nervous system in some way.

Sleep is not an inactive state. The cells (neurons) in our brain remain active, and require as much energy from oxygen as during states of wakefulness. Yet, our muscles are much more relaxed, such that in one form of sleep (REM, or rapid eye movement sleep) muscle tone diminishes to almost zero. As a result, our basal metabolism may fall by 20% to 30%, and our heart rate as low as 20 below our normal resting rate.

REM sleep is the state necessary for dreaming. Renee Nell has speculated that "we inhale thoughts, ideas, impressions, during our waking life. The dream is the exhaling, the digestive process, of these experiences."[78]

Our need for an appropriate amount of sleep for overall health is indicated in the research of E. Cuyler Hammond in an epidemiological study of over one million persons.[79] People with less than 7 and more than 8 hours of sleep were found in his study to have a higher mortality than those with approximately 7 or 8 hours of sleep.

Meditation

Whereas Aikido and physical conditioning stress action and discipline, meditation is more passive, a "deprogramming" of the mind. Meditation is not a religion, despite its eastern origins. It is essentially a technique for attaining a state of deep passivity, deep relaxation, combined with a heightened awareness.

In contrast to the usual swirl of thoughts concerned with yesterday's regrets and tomorrow's problems, meditation is a quiet observing attitude, which "keeps close contact with the here-and-now of experience. Thoughts are not prevented but are allowed to pass without elaboration." It is not a trance, nor sleep, but a deep physical relaxation in which we let go of our usual thought process. Requiring typically two periods of 15 to 20 minutes per day, it proves to be amazingly simple to practice, as well as to learn.

Dr. Herbert Benson of Harvard University has conducted studies on a number of meditative approaches. He believes that twice-a-day meditation offers more rest than an entire night's sleep. In one study, insomniacs who required an average of 75 minutes to fall asleep before transcendental meditation (TM), after only 30 days of TM practice fall asleep in an average of 18 minutes.[80]

Other studies have shown that alcoholics drink less, smokers stop smoking, and drug users kick the habit.

How does meditation produce these remarkable results? According to the founder of TM, Marharishi Yogi, meditation uses the natural tendency of the mind to move always in the direction of greater happiness. All of life exhibits this tendency to move toward greater fulfillment, he explains. TM merely sets the direction. Yet TM meditators do not employ concentration or contemplation. The meditator merely relaxes, allowing the mind to pursue its natural development, while the meditator gently repeats his *mantra*. The mantra is a word with sound but no meaning; its function is to enhance rest and awareness. During the process all thoughts and feelings are observed and accepted.

Although TM, as now established, requires a teacher and a fee, you can learn a number of techniques on your own with a few simple written instructions.

A very simple technique, which should especially appeal to Westerners, has been described by Chaudhuri and derives from Yoga:

The ... approach begins with the resolve to do nothing, to think nothing, to make no effort of one's own, to relax completely and let go of one's mind and body ... stepping out of the stream of ever-changing ideas and feelings which your mind is, watch the on-rush of the stream. Refuse to be submerged in the current. Changing the metaphor, it may be said, watch your ideas, feelings and wishes fly across the mental firmament like a flock of birds. Let them fly freely. Just keep a watch. Don't allow the birds to carry you off into the clouds.

In a Zen meditative practice the individual is simply instructed to count his breaths from one to ten, then repeat. A specified procedure was outlined by Goleman.

Find a quiet place with a straight-back chair. Sit in any comfortable position with your back straight. Close your eyes. Bring your full attention to the movement of your breath as it enters and leaves your nostrils. Don't follow the breath into your lungs or out into the air. Keep your focus at the nostrils, noting the full passage of each in and out breath, from its beginning to its end. Each time your mind wanders to other thoughts, or is caught by background noises, bring your attention back to the easy, natural rhythm of your breathing. Don't try to control the breath; simply be aware of it. Fast or slow, shallow or deep, the nature of the breath does not matter; your total attention to it is what counts. If you have trouble keeping your mind on the breath, count each inhalation and exhalation up to 10, then start over again. Meditate for 20 minutes; set a timer, or peek at your watch occasionally. Doing so won't break your concentration. For the best results, meditate regularly, twice a day, at the same time and place.[81]

After you are able to concentrate completely, progress to a more advanced exercise in which you focus on the process of breathing itself. According to Naranjo and Ornstein, the practitioner then "thinks about nothing but the movement of the air within himself, the air reaching his nose, going down into his lungs, remaining in his lungs, and finally the process of exhalation."[82]

Thus, we can see that meditation is as natural as breathing and may be the most effective means for relaxation. And there are an increasing number of scientific studies in universities which have demonstrated its positive physiological effects. Try it and see for yourself.

Gestalt Therapy

A characteristic of the neurotic person is the inability to feel. Experiencing is resisted because it might cause too much pain. According to the Gestaltists, we are healthy when we are in touch with these feelings, with ourselves, and with our environment. We are unhealthy to the extent we repress our feelings and thoughts. "The regaining of health is to restore the awareness we have lost," explains Dr. Joel Latner.[83]

When we repress our feelings, we can still feel their impulse to be expressed; if strong enough we may even feel we are choking on them or a "bursting of excitement." We can sense this impulse to complete the feeling, the thought, the action that is called for in this situation, in this moment. Repressing these impulses is experienced as anxiety; or when the repression is more severe, as depression; or, still more severe, as muscle tension.

The therapy of Gestalt is a group of exercises that help us to sense fully again; to sharpen our awareness of inner and outer stimuli. One of the advantages of Gestalt therapy is that to a large extent it is a "do-it-yourself" psychotherapy. It helps to have a trained therapist (they work mostly with groups), but we can perform these exercises and sharpen our awareness in the privacy of our own homes. It works if we work.

Common Thrust of All Methods

If we look at the causes of our tensions we begin to understand the common dynamics behind all of the above described disciplines. When we experience physical or emotional pain, if not discharged through the complete experiencing of an appropriate emotion, it tends to be locked up in our mind and body. That is, if we cannot consciously experience the appropriate emotion it is stored in our subconscious and tends to "replay" in some disguised form, such as anxiety, or some psychosomatic illness. These locked-in emotions will block us from the free functioning of our physical, emotional and mental capacities, unless we can find some way to re-experience the traumatic event, to restore to consciousness these hidden memories. Psychoanalysis tries to do this through "free association"; Gestalt therapy by promoting "organismic self-regulation"; Scientology by "auditing"; meditation by a mind-body state which allows our automatic self restorative processes to clear away the hangups. Institutes, such as Esalen in California and Arica in New York City, utilize a blend of physical conditioning, meditation, and interpersonal approaches.

The optimal management of tension will probably require more than the use of a single technique. Nevertheless, beginning with a simple technique can lessen our tensions and anxieties, and can encourage us to search further into pathways which promise greater rewards—total release and attainment of optimal functioning.

Dedicated involvement in a single technique frequently becomes the first step that generates the excitement and confidence necessary to pursue even higher pathways to growth.

Part Six:
Integrating Your
Different Dimensions

23
Breaking Your Chains

A major theme of this book is that destructive living habits are the principle causes of the disabilities and deaths in our society. It follows that the most effective way to prevent or control the diseases in question is to change our faulty living habits. Changing deeply ingrained habits is not an easy task for anyone but gratifying results can be achieved by the proper motivation, methods, and commitment. In this chapter practical techniques for habit-changing will be described.

Will you try an experiment with us to demonstrate the power of a habit? First, simply fold your arms. Next, note which hand is on top of an arm and which is tucked under an arm. Now, reverse the manner in which you fold your arms so that the opposite hand is on top and the other tucked under. Does this feel awkward? Most people find that the second, their non-habitual way, is uncomfortable, unpleasant, and they are not likely to repeat it. In contrast, our habitual way of folding our arms or any other habit feels natural, pleasant, and we perform it automatically.

We have countless habits: the way we tie our shoelaces, the way we shave, eat, greet a friend, or react to stress. Many of these habits are useful. We develop them at some period in our lives because they satisfied a need or situation. Through repetitions they became automatic, and it is no longer necessary to think through the steps of even very complicated acts such as driving a car. We are able to devote our mind to other matters.

Some of these habits become undesirable to us as we or our circumstances change. Eating 4000 calories a day may be appropriate for a 240-lb college football player, but is a health hazard later on. Cigarette smoking is a habit practiced by millions that is a proven danger to health and a $20,000 direct expense over a lifetime of two packs a day. It is even more costly to the habitual smoker who develops a heart attack, cancer, or emphysema, to which smoking makes one much more susceptible. Of equal importance to us are the positive habits we should develop such as a regular exercise program, or habits of study, and self-development.

Fortunately, the same principles apply to the making of desirable habits as to breaking of undesirable ones. Although there are many useful techniques of habit change, we will confine ourselves to one of the most effective ones, namely, "behavior modification." Scientists who specialize in this approach claim substantial success in a wide variety of habits.

What is "behavior modification," and how does it work? Actually, the basic premise is quite simple: "If you do something and are rewarded, you will do it again. If you do something and are punished, you will be motivated not to do it again." If you decide to apply this technique, you will need to acquire an understanding of how habits are formed and changed.

Consider the smoker. He lights up in response to some urge (an internal stimulus) or some circumstance or place (an external stimulus) in which he is accustomed to smoke. The internal stimulus may be internal tensions; a circumstance may be sitting down in one's favorite chair to watch TV. Psychologists say these stimuli (internal urges or external circumstances) become associated (bonded) with the response of smoking if the response is immediately rewarded (or reinforced) in some way.

And the bond (link) is weakened if the response is quickly followed by punishment. We know that in the case of smokers these bonds become very strong. This is because each smoke is quickly rewarded by the relief of tension, which is a powerful reward, indeed. For a two-pack-a-day smoker, this reward strengthens his cigarette habit forty times a day!

How do we break such habits? The habit bonds can be weakened or eliminated in four ways:

● Eliminate the stimulus situations that are linked with smoking. For example, the smoker could stop sitting in his favorite TV chair where he usually smokes. Unfortunately, smoking is linked to innumerable situations, most of which are unavoidable. Nevertheless, this technique can be quite useful for certain habits.

● Prevent the reward from happening, and thereby eventually weaken the bond. Unfortunately, in the case of smoking and other habits, the reward is built into the response itself (the smoking response reduces tension).

● Link the stimulus with another response, a response incompatible with the act of smoking. Many ex-smokers have used this technique successfully. For example, when they feel the urge to smoke they substitute a chewing gum response for the smoking response. The chewing gum response is intrinsically rewarded by a pleasurable taste and, possibly tension relief, and may form a stronger habit than smoking. An unlimited number of harmless or health-promoting activities (responses) can be arranged to follow the urge to smoke with rewards to reinforce the new response. This is the technique most used in behavior modification.

● Punish the response instead of allowing the reward. Some systems to break the smoking habit use this technique. The cigarettes may be made sour, induce nausea, or result in some other form of punishment. Though such approaches may beem repugnant, if applied skillfully, and especially if self-administered, they may be very effective. One simple technique is to carry a rubber band around your wrist and snap it whenever you violate your plan.

Let us now illustrate these princples through a sequence of steps in the breaking of the smoking habit:

Step 1: You will need a strong commitment to carry out the behavior modification procedure. One effective way to examine your commitment is to draw up a pro and con list. Draw a line down the center of a page: on the left, write the reasons you want to quit smoking, and on the right the reasons that are encouraging you to continue smoking. The more thought you give to this list, the greater your insight into the forces that motivate you to change your habit or to perpetuate it. Examine this list every day and add to it as you think of additional pros and cons.

Step 2: Devise a reward system that you will use to reinforce your new nonsmoking habit. This is perhaps the most critical step, as the items or events you select as your reward for correct response must in fact be an appealing reward to you. The strength of this reward establishes the power of the habit change system.

To help you identify rewards, list all the possible things you enjoy such as attending a sports event, movie, a play, or a concert, purchasing a book or records, a camera, new clothes or jewelry, vacation trips, etc. Be as specific as you can in making the list.

As an example you might establish your reward system in the following way:

• For each perfect day (no cigarettes) place a dollar into a special savings account. Because you are not buying cigarettes, nor do you have other costs associated with cigarettes, this reward system pays for itself.

• For each perfect month, an additional 10 perfect days are allotted to this bank account.

• For every X number of rules adhered to on non-perfect days, $1.00 is allotted.

This savings account can be used for whatever the habit-changer wishes. To ensure that your selected reward is a real reward, it is important that you pick things or events that you would not otherwise allow yourself.

Step 3: Follow a sequence of rules that progressively shape a nonsmoking habit pattern. The following system of rules have been found to be especially effective: Each rule represents two days. That is, follow rule one for two days. Then, circle the rule when you have correctly adhered to it on day one, and a second circle on day two. Next, follow rule one and rule two for the next two days, and so on. If you do not adhere to a given rule for two consecutive days, remain at that rule until you do.

1. Buy only one pack at a time.
2. Always refuse any cigarette offered.
3. Never smoke your first cigarette until after breakfast.
4. Every day put aside the exact amount of money you've saved by smoking less.
5. Stop smoking outdoors and in bed.
6. Don't keep your cigarette in your hand. Put it down after each puff.
7. Don't smoke while driving.

8. Wait two minutes before lighting each cigarette.

9. Don't smoke while waiting to eat.

10. Smoke each cigarette just halfway.

11. If you feel the urge to smoke, look at your watch and wait five minutes.

12. Increase the time before lighting each cigarette to ten minutes.

13. Get up after a meal without a cigarette and immediately busy yourself.

14. Extinguish each cigarette after the first puff, then relight.

15. Smoke only at a specific place.

16. If you have to smoke, do only that. Don't read, watch TV, drink, work, eat, etc.

17. Don't smoke in the presence of others.

18. Try to stop inhaling.

19. Don't smoke during working hours.

This system works if you work. Never mind if some of the rules appear silly or inconsequential. You will soon find that they are in fact remarkably effective. You must decide to be exacting about your adherence to the system. It does require a firm commitment and honesty to one's self.

Many habits can be managed in the same manner. Robbins and Fisher [84] offer this sound general advice:

• Don't be afraid of relapses. At the beginning you may forget or just fail to perform the new habit. It's going to happen, so don't worry about it. Just remember, the more often you repeat the habit, the easier it is to learn it.

• Let people around you know what your plans are: the more help you have, the better.

• Constant reminders are beneficial. Provide yourself with plenty of reminders. You are trying to teach yourself something new, and it will take time for it to become ingrained. Use little signs, messages, anything to remind you to do what you want to get into the habit of doing.

• Don't be too alarmed if you are not truthful with yourself at first. Eventually, most people start being accurate. They realize it is not smart to fool oneself.

• Make all rewards and punishments simple. Remember they serve an important purpose. They are reminders as well as motivators. Don't make them so powerful or outlandish that you are always thinking about them or afraid of the consequences.

- Make sure that the reinforcements follow the time period during which the habit should have taken place. It does no good to penalize yourself three hours after you forget to do something.

- Don't drop your conditioning system until the habit is deeply ingrained. Even though you have established a habit quickly, keep using the system for at least a month. We cannot give you a 100% guarantee that this behavior modification system will work for you on a habit you want to change. But we believe you are likely to be very pleasantly surprised and rewarded if you give it a try.

24
Whole Person
Concept

When health is absent, wisdom cannot reveal itself, art cannot become manifest, strength cannot fight, wealth becomes useless, and intelligence cannot be applied.

Herophilus,
Physician of Alexandria

Since ancient times, philosophers have proposed that man was one in body, mind, and spirit. Whatever affected the body would influence the emotions and even our thoughts. Man does not consist simply of fragments of organs, attitudes, beliefs, and feelings. These elements act in concert, such that the whole is greater than the sum of the parts. We begin to appreciate these interrelationships when an injury, a threatening situation, or a beautiful scene transforms in a moment our thinking, feeling, and behavior.

Because we are mind as well as body, we will not attain optimal health solely through attention to a series of physical exercises. Nor will we completely master any single fitness practice in isolation from other life habits. Movement toward health is more a summation of numerous small insights, more a journey than a leap.

This realization can be disillusioning to those who seek a panacea, a singular solution, to their life difficulties. But belief in the wholeness of man, of the interdependence of our parts can be heartening as well. Wholeness means that any constructive act, however small, will have some measure of beneficial effect throughout the smallest reaches of our being.

In this respect our journey toward optimal health will begin with small positive steps. In this way any goal can be reached, no matter how remote or difficult. What we can accomplish is limited only by our belief in what is possible, and by our willingness to commit to that first step.

This book has offered a number of concepts and health practices. But neither understanding nor growth can occur simply through an intellectual grasp of these ideas. Real understanding is a result of doing, not reading. Comprehension is not enough, it requires an act of courage, a willingness to commit to a line of action and see the truth of it for oneself. What will result from action will be insight and application of health practices in accord with your unique capacities and interests.

Some may reject this comprehensive view as being too involved. "All I really need to do is . . ." We Americans pride ourselves on being practical. We want results fast. "Got a headache? Take an aspirin." Never mind that the headache may represent signals from our body calling for awareness of a deeper problem. Rather we are inclined to apply drugs that dull these signals, in order that we might hurry back to our self-destructive behavior. Try this test on yourself. If you were to learn that your blood pressure was too high, which solution would be most appealing to you?:

• A new drug that lowers blood pressure
• Drug treatment plus a program to lose weight
• Both of the above, plus a willingness to re-examine your entire lifestyle, and make changes in your habits of exercise, eating, working, use of leisure and rest.

The first two solutions are bound to be inadequate. One is not even likely to be successful in permanent changes in weight, without major lifestyle changes. Yet we know that hypertension is a serious problem. So are such diseases as diabetes, heart disease, and cancer, all greatly affected by lifestyle. These are life or death matters.

Health Is Your Responsibility

To whom can we look for help? There are physicians who take the view that to give the patient the full picture will alarm him and aggravate the problem, or that people won't change their behavior anyway, or that a full explanation takes a prohibitively long time. Our view is that health is mainly the responsibility of the individual. Of course he needs to have all the facts and sound, professional and intelligible advice as well. Then the commitment is up to him.

Broader solutions to degenerative diseases are more in keeping with the nature of these diseases. We can identify a micro-organism as the specific cause of an infectious disease. In contrast, degenerative diseases, such as cardiovascular diseases, result from a long list of risk factors operating over many years, which in turn is the result of failure to apply the health-fitness practices described in this book. We forge our diseases link by link, through decades of improper habits of eating, exercise, rest, mental attitudes, and human relationships. There is no single cause of coronary heart disease—it is the result of the way we live, day by day, year after year.

How, then, can you as a whole person, strive toward optimal health? The first step is to consider the dimensions of the person that interweave to form the whole. The early philosophers described man as consisting of body, mind, and spirit. We prefer a conception that employs six dimensions.

The Sixth Dimension

1. Physical. Development of our physical dimension, our body, provides us with a foundation of energy with which to pursue our goals and withstand the stresses of life. There are two skills (and fields of knowledge) to master this dimension: fitness and leisure. This book is an attempt to convey some of this crucial knowledge.

2. Emotional. Growth in our emotional dimension leads us toward a confident self-image, a high self-esteem. Much progress has been made in recent years by behavioral scientists to develop concepts and skills the nonprofessional person can use to develop in this dimension. Examples of such techniques are transactional analysis, Gestalt therapy, meditation, rational therapy, various awareness building techniques, and the "positive image" approaches. Since our self esteem is closely related to our esteem of others and with intimacy, we might add encounter group techniques and similar interpersonal disciplines.

3. Intellectual. Our intellectual dimension is the means by which we assimilate the knowledge of our culture. We reach the great teachers through the capacity to read, listen, and observe, and problem-solve skillfully. The finest teachers who have ever lived are available to us through books, providing we have mastered the skill and art of effective reading.

4. *Social.* Man is a social being. The development of all that is significant about man: our language and our culture, is the result of collaboration with others. Some of our greatest enjoyments and life meanings are found in our associations with others. Therefore, our social dimension, our interpersonal skills, are integral to our wholeness.

5. *Vocational.* Our vocational dimension involves the skills with which we meet our economic needs and obligations. We spend the larger portion of our waking hours seeking mastery over some technical or professional vocation. For most of us this need is primary. It is essential to our survival and is tied closely to our concept of self-worth as well.

6. *Spiritual.* Finally, when man asks the basic questions: Who am I? why am I here? where am I going? he expresses a deep searching for the meaning of his existence. Most societies assume a deity or deities and believe that man stands in some special relationship to them. Our hunger for the meaning of life may be greater than our hunger for food. Some seek through spiritual means the wisdom to guide all aspects of their life, including their physical health. They may even believe physical health is attainable directly through spiritual insight or grace.

We see every one of these dimensions as pathways toward wholeness, pathways that contribute to optimal health. One may stress one or the other according to his temperament and upbringing. However, from the standpoint of health, we propose one fundamental principle:

Growth in any dimension will have a constructive impact on all other dimensions. Conversely, any deterioration of any one dimension will, in some degree, injure all other dimensions.

The fit body, for example, promotes an emotional sense of well-being; illness generates fear, self doubt, despair. We can see these kinds of interconnections extending to other dimensions: the high energy reserve of a fit body will support perseverance in intellectual endeavors, aggressive pursuance of vocational ambitions, and perhaps even a vibrant receptivity to spiritual progress.

Scientists are now discovering that an emotional experience

or pain is likewise locked in some subtle, but specific, way in the muscles. In this way our emotional experiences become locked within our memories and in our musculature, affecting even our physical posture. All of our life habits are assimilated into our whole being and will reflect in our expression and our bearing.

Each dimension has an impact on each other dimension. Our dimensions act as one; therefore, we cannot without eventual penalty, allow any to degenerate. We share with our creator the privilege of creating ourselves.

Our view is that constructive steps toward optimal health will reverberate through all the dimensions of our person, and also significantly touch the lives of those around us. Though not a light responsibility, neither is it an overwhelming one. Optimal health-fitness, an attainable goal, is evidenced by many who have reached their goals. And it is one that we will be able to see, feel, and believe as tangible results inevitably follow a sound health-fitness program. Ultimately, it is your decision, your responsibility, your commitment.

We hope this book will contribute in some way to your journey. We wish you long life filled with joy and health-fitness for the years ahead.

Appendices

Appendix A: Nutritive Value of Foods

	Measure	Weight	Food Energy	Protein	Fat	Carbohydrate	Calcium	Potassium	Vitamin B$_2$	Vitamin B$_1$	Vitamin B$_6$	Vitamin C
		grams	cal.	grams	grams	grams	mg.	mg.	mg.	mg.	mg.	mg.
DAIRY PRODUCTS												
CHEESE												
Cheddar, shredded	1 cup	113	455	28	37	1	815	111	0.03	0.42	0.1	0
Cottage cheese	1 cup	225	235	23	10	6	135	190	0.05	0.37	0.3	Trace
Cream cheese	1 oz.	28	100	2	10	—	—	34	Trace	0.06	Trace	0
Pasteurized American cheese	1 oz.	28	105	6	6	Trace	174	46	0.01	0.10	Trace	0
CREAM												
Half-and-half	1 tbsp.	15	20	Trace	2	1	16	19	0.01	0.02	Trace	Trace
Cream, sour	1 tbsp.	12	25	Trace	3	1	14	17	Trace	0.02	Trace	Trace
MILK												
Whole	1 cup	244	150	8	8	11	291	370	0.09	0.40	0.2	2
Lowfat (2%)	1 cup	244	120	8	5	12	297	377	0.10	0.40	0.2	2
Nonfat (skim)	1 cup	245	85	8	Trace	12	302	406	0.09	0.37	0.2	2
ICE CREAM												
Hardened	1 cup	133	270	5	115	32	176	257	0.05	0.33	0.1	1
Soft (frozen custard)	1 cup	173	375	7	23	38	236	338	0.08	0.45	0.2	1
YOGURT												
Fruit-flavored	8 oz.	227	230	10	3	42	343	439	0.08	0.40	0.2	1

Food												
Plain	8 oz.	227	145	12	4	16	415	531	0.10	0.49	0.3	2
EGGS												
Fried in butter	1 egg	46	85	5	6	1	26	58	0.03	0.13	Trace	0
Hard-cooked, shell removed	1 egg	50	80	6	6	1	28	65	0.04	0.14	Trace	0
Scrambled (milk added in butter; also omelet	1 egg	64	95	6	7	1	47	85	0.04	0.16	Trace	0
FATS AND OILS												
Butter	1 tbsp.	14	100	Trace	12	Trace	3	4	Trace	Trace	Trace	0
Vegetable shortening	1 tbsp.	13	110	0	13	0	0	0	0	0	0	0
Margarine	1 tbsp.	14	100	Trace	12	Trace	0	4	Trace	Trace	Trace	0
Corn oil	1 tbsp.	14	120	0	14	0	0	0	0	0	0	0
Soybean-cottonseed oil blend, hydrogenated	1 tbsp.	14	120	0	14	0	0	0	0	0	0	0
FISH, MEAT, AND POULTRY												
FISH												
Haddock, breaded, fried	3 oz.	85	140	17	5	5	34	296	0.03	0.06	2.7	2
Ocean perch, breaded, fried	1 fillet	85	195	16	11	6	28	242	0.10	0.10	1.6	—
Tuna, canned (in oil, drained)	3 oz.	85	170	24	7	0	7	—	0.04	0.10	10.1	—
MEAT												
Bacon, broiled or fried, crisp	2 slices	15	85	4	8	Trace	2	35	0.08	0.05	0.8	—
Beef, braised, simmered, or roasted	3 oz.	85	245	23	16	0	10	184	0.04	0.18	3.6	—
Ground beef, broiled	2.9 oz.	82	235	20	17	0	9	221	0.07	0.17	4.4	—
Roast, oven cooked	3 oz.	85	375	17	33	0	8	189	0.05	0.13	3.1	—
Steak, sirloin, broiled	3 oz.	85	330	20	27	0	9	220	0.05	0.15	4.0	—

Measure	Weight (cal.)	Food Energy (grams)	Protein (grams)	Fat (grams)	Carbohydrate (mg.)	Calcium (mg.)	Potassium (mg.)	Vitamin B2 (mg.)	Vitamin B1 (mg.)	Vitamin B6 (mg.)	Vitamin C (mg.)
Lamb											
Chop, broiled — 3.1 oz.	89	360	18	32	0	8	200	0.11	0.19	4.1	—
Leg, roasted — 3 oz.	85	235	22	16	0	9	241	0.13	0.23	4.7	—
Liver, fried — 3 oz.	85	195	22	9	5	9	323	0.22	3.56	14.0	23
Ham, roasted — 3 oz.	85	245	18	19	0	8	199	0.40	0.15	3.1	—
Pork											
Chop — 2.7 oz.	78	305	19	25	0	9	216	0.75	0.22	4.5	—
Roast, oven cooked — 3 oz.	85	310	21	24	0	9	233	0.78	0.22	4.8	—
Sausages											
Bologna — 1 slice	28	85	3	8	Trace	2	65	0.05	0.06	0.7	—
Brown and serve — 1 link	17	70	3	6	Trace	—	—	—	—	—	—
Frankfurter, cooked — 1 ea.	56	170	7	15	1	3	—	0.08	0.11	1.4	—
Pork link, cooked — 1 link	13	60	2	6	Trace	1	35	0.10	0.04	0.5	—
Salami, cooked type — 1 slice	28	90	5	7	Trace	3	—	0.07	0.07	1.2	—
Veal, cutlet — 3 oz.	85	185	23	9	0	9	258	0.06	0.21	4.6	—
POULTRY											
Chicken, cooked											
Drumstick, fried — 1.3 oz.	38	90	12	4	Trace	6	—	0.03	0.15	2.7	—
Half-broiler, broiled — 6.2 oz.	176	240	42	7	0	16	483	0.09	0.35	15.5	—

Turkey, roasted, flesh without skin

Food												
Dark meat	4 pcs.	85	175	26	7	0	—	338	0.03	0.20	3.6	—
Light meat	2 pcs.	85	150	28	3	0	—	349	0.04	0.12	9.4	—

FRUITS AND FRUIT PRODUCTS

Food												
Apples, raw, unpeeled	1 ea.	138	80	Trace	1	20	10	152	0.04	0.03	0.1	6
Apricots												
Raw	3	107	55	1	Trace	14	18	301	0.03	0.04	0.6	11
Canned	1 cup	258	220	2	Trace	57	28	604	0.05	0.05	1.0	10
Avocados, raw, whole	1 ea.	216	370	5	37	13	22	1303	0.24	0.43	3.5	30
Banana	1 ea.	119	100	1	Trace	26	10	440	0.06	0.07	0.8	12
Grapefruit, medium	1/2 ea.	241	50	1	Trace	13	20	166	0.05	0.02	0.2	44
Grapes, seedless	10	50	35	Trace	Trace	9	6	87	0.03	0.02	0.2	2
Lemonade, diluted	1 cup	248	105	Trace	Trace	28	2	40	0.01	0.02	0.2	17
Melons												
Cantaloupe	1/2 ea.	477	80	2	Trace	20	38	682	0.11	0.08	1.6	90
Honeydew	1/10 ea.	226	50	1	Trace	11	21	374	0.06	0.04	0.9	34
Oranges	1 ea.	131	65	1	Trace	16	54	263	0.13	0.05	0.5	66
Orange juice, frozen, diluted	1 cup	249	120	2	Trace	29	25	503	0.23	0.03	0.9	120
Papayas, raw	1 cup	140	55	1	Trace	14	28	328	0.06	0.06	0.4	78
Peaches, whole	1 ea.	100	40	1	Trace	10	9	202	0.02	0.05	1.0	7
Pears, raw, with skin, cored	1 ea.	164	100	1	1	25	13	213	0.03	0.07	0.2	7
Pineapple												
Raw, diced	1 cup	155	80	1	Trace	21	26	226	0.14	0.05	0.3	26
Canned	1 slice	105	80	Trace	Trace	20	12	101	0.08	0.02	0.2	7
Pineapple juice, unsweetened	1 cup	250	140	1	Trace	34	38	373	0.13	0.05	0.5	80
Raisins, seedless	1 cup	145	420	4	Trace	112	90	1106	0.16	0.12	0.7	1

	Measure	Weight	Food Energy	Protein	Fat	Carbohydrate	Calcium	Potassium	Vitamin B2	Vitamin B1	Vitamin B6	Vitamin C
	grams	cal.	grams	grams	grams	mg.	mg.	mg.	mg.	mg.	mg.	mg.
Strawberries, raw, whole berries	1 cup	149	55	1	1	13	31	244	0.04	0.10	0.9	88
GRAIN PRODUCTS												
BREADS												
Cracked-wheat bread	1 slice	25	65	2	1	13	22	34	0.08	0.06	0.08	Trace
French, enriched	1 slice	35	100	3	1	19	15	32	0.14	0.08	1.2	Trace
Rye bread	1 slice	25	60	2	Trace	13	19	36	0.07	0.05	0.7	0
White bread, enriched	1 slice	23	65	2	1	12	22	28	0.09	0.06	0.8	Trace
Whole-wheat bread	1 slice	25	60	3	1	12	25	68	0.06	0.03	0.7	Trace
BREAKFAST CEREALS												
Oatmeal or rolled oats	1 cup	240	130	5	2	23	22	146	0.19	0.05	0.2	0
Bran flakes (40% bran)	1 cup	35	105	4	1	28	19	137	0.41	0.49	4.1	12
Cornflakes	1 cup	25	95	2	Trace	21	—	30	0.29	0.35	2.9	9
Wheat, puffed	1 cup	15	55	2	Trace	12	4	51	0.08	0.03	1.2	0
Wheat, shredded, plain biscuit	1	25	90	2	1	20	11	87	0.06	0.03	1.1	0
OTHER GRAIN PRODUCTS												
Wheat germ	1 tbsp.	6	25	2	1	3	3	57	0.11	0.05	0.3	1
Cornmeal, whole-ground	1 cup	122	435	11	5	90	24	346	0.46	0.13	2.4	0
Crackers												
Graham	2	14	55	1	1	10	6	55	0.02	0.08	0.5	0

Food	Measure											
Saltines	4	11	50	1	1	8	2	13	0.05	0.05	0.4	0
Macaroni, enriched, cooked	1 cup	140	155	5	1	32	11	85	0.20	0.11	1.5	0
Pancakes (4-in. diam.)	1 cake	27	60	2	2	9	58	42	0.04	0.06	0.2	Trace
Rice, white, enriched	1 cup	205	225	4	Trace	50	21	57	0.23	0.02	2.1	0
Barley (pearled, light, uncooked)	1 cup	200	700	16	2	158	32	320	0.24	0.10	6.2	0
Wheat flour												
Sifted	1 cup	115	420	12	1	88	18	109	0.74	0.46	6.1	0
Whole wheat	1 cup	120	400	16	2	85	49	444	0.66	0.14	5.2	0

LEGUMES (DRY), NUTS, AND SEEDS

Food	Measure											
Almonds, shelled	1 cup	130	775	24	70	25	304	1005	0.31	1.20	4.6	Trace
Beans, cooked												
Great northern	1 cup	180	210	14	1	38	90	749	0.25	0.13	1.3	0
Navy	1 cup	190	225	15	1	40	95	790	0.27	0.13	1.3	0
Lima, cooked, drained	1 cup	190	260	16	1	49	55	1163	0.25	0.11	1.3	—
Coconut meat, fresh	1 cup	80	275	3	28	8	10	205	0.04	0.02	0.4	2
Lentils, whole, cooked	1 cup	200	210	16	Trace	39	50	498	0.14	0.12	1.2	0
Peanuts, roasted in oil, salted	1 cup	144	840	37	72	27	107	971	0.46	0.19	24.8	0
Peanut butter	1 tbsp.	16	95	4	8	3	9	100	0.02	0.02	2.4	0
Peas, split, dry, cooked	1 cup	200	230	16	1	42	22	592	0.30	0.18	1.8	—

SUGARS

Food	Measure											
Honey	1 tbsp.	21	65	Trace	0	17	1	11	Trace	0.01	0.1	Trace
Sugars												
Brown	1 cup	220	820	0	0	212	187	757	0.02	0.07	0.4	0
White	1 cup	200	770	0	0	199	0	6	0	0	0	0

VEGETABLES

	Measure (grams)	Weight (cal.)	Food Energy (grams)	Protein (grams)	Fat (grams)	Carbohydrate (mg.)	Calcium (mg.)	Potassium (mg.)	Vitamin B₂ (mg.)	Vitamin B₁ (mg.)	Vitamin B₆ (mg.)	Vitamin C (mg.)
Asparagus, cooked	1 cup	145	30	3	Trace	5	30	265	0.23	0.26	2.0	38
Beans												
Lima, frozen, cooked, drained,	1 cup	180	210	13	Trace	40	63	709	0.16	0.09	2.2	22
Green, cooked, drained, from raw	1 cup	125	30	2	Trace	7	63	189	0.09	0.11	0.6	15
Bean sprouts, cooked, drained	1 cup	125	35	4	Trace	7	21	195	0.11	0.13	0.9	8
Beets, cooked, drained, peeled, whole 2 in. diam.	2 ea.	100	30	1	Trace	7	14	208	0.03	0.04	0.3	6
Broccoli, cooked, drained												
Fresh	1 cup	155	40	5	Trace	7	136	414	0.14	0.31	1.2	140
Frozen, chopped	1 cup	185	50	5	1	9	100	392	0.11	0.22	0.9	105
Brussels sprouts, cooked, drained	1 cup	155	55	7	1	10	50	423	0.12	0.22	1.2	135
Cabbage												
Raw	1 cup	90	20	1	Trace	5	44	210	0.05	0.05	0.3	42
Cooked, drained	1 cup	145	30	2	Trace	6	64	236	0.06	0.06	0.4	48
Carrots												
Raw	1 ea.	72	30	1	Trace	7	27	246	0.04	0.04	0.4	6
Cooked, drained	1 cup	155	50	1	Trace	11	51	344	0.08	0.08	0.8	9
Cauliflower												
Raw	1 cup	115	31	3	Trace	6	29	339	0.13	0.12	0.8	90

Food	Measure											
Cooked from raw	1 cup	125	30	3	Trace	5	26	258	0.11	0.10	0.8	69
Cooked from frozen	1 cup	180	30	3	Trace	6	31	373	0.07	0.09	0.7	74
Celery	1 stalk	40	5	Trace	Trace	2	16	136	0.01	0.01	0.1	4
Corn												
Cooked from raw	1 ear	140	70	2	1	16	2	151	0.09	0.08	1.1	7
Cooked from frozen	1 cup	165	130	5	1	31	5	304	0.15	0.10	2.5	8
Canned, cream style	1 cup	256	210	5	2	51	8	248	0.08	0.13	2.6	13
Canned, whole kernel	1 cup	210	175	5	1	43	6	204	0.06	0.13	2.3	11
Cucumber	6 large	28	5	Trace	Trace	1	7	45	0.01	0.01	0.1	3
Lettuce												
Butter, leaves	2	15	Trace	Trace	Trace	Trace	5	40	0.01	0.01	Trace	1
Iceberg pieces	1 cup	55	5	Trace	Trace	2	11	96	0.03	0.03	0.2	3
Mushrooms, raw	1 cup	70	20	2	Trace	3	4	290	0.07	0.32	2.9	2
Onions												
Raw, chopped	1 cup	170	65	3	Trace	15	46	267	0.05	0.07	0.3	17
Cooked	1 cup	210	60	3	Trace	14	50	231	0.06	0.06	0.4	15
Green	6 ea.	30	15	Trace	Trace	3	12	69	0.02	0.01	0.1	8
Peas, green												
Canned whole	1 cup	170	150	8	1	29	44	163	0.15	0.10	1.4	14
Frozen	1 cup	160	110	8	Trace	19	30	216	0.43	0.14	2.7	21
Potatoes												
Baked	1 ea.	156	145	4	Trace	33	14	782	0.15	0.07	2.7	31
Boiled	1 ea.	135	90	3	Trace	20	8	385	0.12	0.05	1.6	22
Pumpkin, canned	1 cup	245	80	2	1	19	61	588	0.07	0.12	1.5	12
Radishes, raw	4 ea.	18	5	Trace	Trace	1	5	58	0.01	0.01	0.1	5

	Measure	Weight	Food Energy	Protein	Fat	Carbohydrate	Calcium	Potassium	Vitamin B$_2$	Vitamin B$_1$	Vitamin B$_6$	Vitamin C
	grams	cal.	grams	grams	grams	mg.	mg.	mg.	mg.	mg.	mg.	mg.
Spinach												
Raw, chopped	1 cup	55	15	2	Trace	2	51	259	0.06	0.11	0.3	28
Cooked from raw	1 cup	180	40	5	1	6	167	583	0.13	0.25	0.9	50
Cooked from frozen	1 cup	205	45	6	1	8	232	683	0.14	0.31	0.8	39
Squash												
Summer	1 cup	210	30	2	Trace	7	53	296	0.11	0.17	1.7	21
Winter	1 cup	205	130	4	1	32	57	945	0.10	0.27	1.4	27
Sweet potatoes	1 ea.	114	160	2	1	37	46	342	0.10	0.08	0.8	25
Tomatoes	1 ea.	135	25	1	Trace	6	16	300	0.07	0.05	0.9	28
Tomato catsup	1 tbsp.	15	15	Trace	Trace	4	3	54	0.01	0.01	0.2	2
Tomato juice, canned	1 glass	182	35	2	Trace	8	13	413	0.09	0.05	1.5	29
Turnips, cooked, diced	1 cup	155	35	1	Trace	8	54	291	0.06	0.08	0.5	34

Note: These figures represent the nutritive value of foods listed in the exact measurements, following traditional cooking methods. For more specific information, consult the product label. Dashes (—) denote lack of reliable data on measurable amounts.

RECOMMENDED DAILY ALLOWANCES

Sex/Age category	Age (yrs.)	Weight (lbs.)	Height (in.)	Food energy (calories)	Protein (grams)	Cal-cium (mg.)	Phos-phorus (mg.)	Iron (mg.)	Vita-min A (Int. units)	Thia-min (mg.)	Ribo-flavin (mg.)	Nia-cin (mg.)	Ascor-bic acid (mg.)
Infants	0–.5	14	24	lb. x 53.2	lb. x 1.0	360	240	10	1,400	0.3	0.4	5	35
	.5–1	20	28	lb. x 49.1	lb. x 0.9	540	400	15	2,000	0.5	0.6	8	35
Children	1–3	28	34	1,300	23	800	800	15	2,000	0.7	0.8	9	40
	4–6	44	44	1,800	30	800	800	10	2,500	0.9	1.1	12	40
	7–10	66	54	2,400	36	800	800	10	3,300	1.2	1.2	16	40
Males	11–14	97	63	2,800	44	1,200	1,200	18	5,000	1.4	1.5	18	45
	15–18	134	69	3,000	54	1,200	1,200	18	5,000	1.5	1.8	20	45
	19–22	147	69	3,000	54	800	800	10	5,000	1.5	1.8	20	45
	23–50	154	69	2,700	56	800	800	10	5,000	1.4	1.6	18	45
	51+	154	69	2,400	56	800	800	10	5,000	1.2	1.5	16	45
Females	11–14	97	62	2,400	44	1,200	1,200	18	4,000	1.2	1.3	16	45
	15–18	119	65	2,100	48	1,200	1,200	18	4,000	1.1	1.4	14	45
	19–22	128	65	2,100	46	800	800	18	4,000	1.1	1.4	14	45
	23–50	128	65	2,000	46	800	800	18	4,000	1.0	1.4	13	45
	51+	128	65	1,800	46	800	800	10	4,000	1.0	1.2	12	45
Pregnant				+300	+30	1,200	1,200	+18	5,000	+0.3	+0.3	+2	60
Lactating				+500	+20	1,200	1,200	18	6,000	+0.3	+0.5	+4	80

Source: Adapted from Recommended Dietary Allowances, 8th ed. (Washington: National Academy of Sciences—National Research Council, 1974).

Appendix B:
Optimal Meals,
Recipes, and Snacks

(Recommended for Optimal, Obesity, Diabetic diets)

LUNCH OR DINNER

1. **Total calories**   399
   4 ounces roast veal
   1 cup steamed zucchini
   large mixed green salad with 1 teaspoon oil and vinegar dressing
   1 cup fresh strawberries
   iced tea or coffee substitute

2. **Total calories**   407
   1 cup beef bouillon
   4 ounces sliced chicken
   1 cup green beans
   1 small dinner roll
   1 large tomato-and-endive salad
   1 medium fresh pear
   tea or coffee substitute

3. **Total calories**   409
   1 cup parsleyed chicken broth
   4 ounces broiled swordfish with lemon
   1 cup fresh asparagus
   1/2 cup pickled beet and Spanish onion salad
   1/2 cup sliced peaches
   4 ounces skim milk

4. **Total calories**   396
   Open-faced hamburger plate
   1/2 large sesame seed bun
   3 ounce beef patty
   1 teaspoon prepared mustard
   tomato slices
   shredded lettuce
   1/2 cup carrot slaw with 2 tablespoons raisins and 1 teaspoon salad
      dressing
   iced tea with lemon

5. **Total calories**   411
   1 cup hot tomato bouillon
   4 ounces turkey salad
   1/2 cup chopped turkey
   1 teaspoon chopped onion

1/2 cup celery
1 teaspoon French dressing
1 small Parker House roll
1 cup fresh broccoli
4 ounces skim milk

6. **Total calories**   **393**
   5 ounces beef bouillon
   1/2 baked Rock Cornish hen
   1/2 cup steamed rice
   1 cup fresh steamed spinach with lemon
   radishes and cucumber slices
   coffee substitute

7. **Total calories**   **397**
   Open-face toasted sandwich
   1 slice wheat bread
   2 ounces American cheese
   1 teaspoon salad mustard
   large tomato salad with 1/2 cup carrot sticks and 1 teaspoon French
      dressing
   1 glass skim milk

8. **Total calories**   **407**
   4 ounces lean roast beef
   1 small baked potato
   1 teaspoon margarine
   1 cup brussels sprouts
   sliced cucumbers in herb vinegar
   hot tea with lemon

Recipes

LEMON BAKED CHICKEN
(145 calories per serving. Makes 4 servings.)
1 frying chicken (2 1/2–3 lbs.) cut into serving pieces
3 tablespoons vegetable oil (corn, safflower or soy)
3 tablespoons fresh lemon juice
1 crushed clove garlic
1/2 teaspoon salt
dash of pepper

Instructions: Arrange chicken in shallow casserole or baking dish. Pour lemon and oil mixture over chicken. Cover and bake until tender, about 45–50 minutes. Uncover casserole the last 10 minutes to allow chicken to brown. Baste occasionally during cooking. Before serving, sprinkle with chopped parsley.

OVEN BAKED FISH
(137 calories per serving. Makes 4 servings.)
1 pound fish fillets or small whole fish
1 cup dry bread crumbs
1/2 cup French dressing (2 parts vegetable oil to 1 part vinegar or lemon
  or lime juice)

Instructions: Preheat oven to 500° (very hot). If frozen fish is used, thaw enough to separate pieces. Dip fish into well seasoned French dressing, then into bread crumbs. Arrange on oiled baking pan. Pour any remaining French dressing over fish. Bake for 10–12 minutes, or until fish flakes easily when tested with a fork.

TUNA MOLD
(117 calories per serving. Makes 5 servings.)
1 envelope unflavored gelatin
1/4 cup cold water
1 1/2 cups boiling water
1/2 teaspoon salt (or 1/8 teaspoon salt substitute)
1–2 drops liquid artificial sweetener
1/4 small green pepper, chopped
1/2 cup chopped stuffed olives
3 tablespoons tarragon or wine vinegar
1 8-oz. can tuna fish, flaked
1/2 red onion, chopped
1/2 cup finely chopped celery

Instructions: Soften gelatin in 1/4-cup cold water. Add boiling water, salt, and liquid sweetener, and stir until gelatin is dissolved. Add the vinegar. Cool mixture in refrigerator until partially congealed. Stir in the flaked tuna and all the chopped vegetables and the olives. Pour into a rinsed mold or into 5 individual fish molds and chill until firmly set. Serve on crisp salad greens.

BUTTERMILK SALAD DRESSING
(11 calories per tablespoon. Makes 1 cup.)
Blend:
1 cup skim milk buttermilk (or low-fat yoghurt)
1 tablespoon chopped onion
1 tablespoon chopped celery
1 tablespoon chopped green pepper
1 tablespoon dietetic chili sauce or catsup
1 tablespoon garlic vinegar
1 teaspoon chopped parsley
1/4 teaspoon salt (or 1/8 teaspoon salt substitute)

Instructions: Allow mixture to stand, after blending, for at least 1 hour to bring out flavor.

Vegetarian Dishes

MACARONI BAKE
(355 calories per serving. Makes 6 servings.)
4 cups cooked macaroni (2 cups uncooked)
1/3 cup chopped onion
1/4 cup margarine
1/4 cup flour
2 cups skim milk
1/2 teaspoon dill weed
1/2 teaspoon dried parsley flakes
1/4 teaspoon pepper
2 cups low fat cottage cheese
1/2 cup bread crumbs

Instructions: Saute onion in margarine just until tender. Stir in flour. Cook 1 minute, stirring constantly. Blend in milk. Cook and stir over medium heat until thick. Add dill weed, parsley flakes, pepper, cottage cheese, and cooked macaroni. Pour into shallow baking dish brushed with margarine. Top with crumbs. Bake at 350° for 45 minutes or until bubbly.

CHIFFON BREAD CRUMBS
(35 calories per tablespoon. Makes about 2 cups.)
1 cup fine dry bread crumbs
1/2 cup Chiffon margarine

Instructions: Measure bread crumbs and margarine into mixing bowl. Blend with pastry blender or fork until thoroughly mixed. Store in refrigerator. May also be used as garnish for any cooked vegetables.

Breads

BISCUITS
(115 calories each. Makes 1 dozen 2 inch biscuits.)
2 cups unsifted all-purpose flour
3 teaspoons baking powder
1 teaspoon salt
1/3 cup margarine
3/4 cup skim milk

Instructions: Measure flour, baking powder, and salt into mixing bowl. Mix well. Cut in margarine with pastry blender or fork until mixture resembles coarse meal. Stir in milk. Mix lightly with fork. Turn out on lightly floured cloth or surface. Knead lightly about 1/2 minute, or until smooth. Roll to 1/2-inch thickness, fold in half, roll out again to 1/2-inch thickness. Cut with a floured 2-inch cutter. Place on ungreased baking sheet. Bake at 450° for 10–12 minutes or until golden brown.

FLUFFY PANCAKES
(85 calories each. Makes 10 4-inch pancakes.)

1 cup unsifted all-purpose flour
1 tablespoon sugar
3 teaspoons baking powder
1/2 teaspoon salt
3 tablespoons margarine
3/4 cup skim milk
2 egg whites, stiffly beaten

Instructions: Measure flour, sugar, baking powder, and salt into mixing bowl. Mix well. Add margarine and break up with fork. Stir in milk only until dry ingredients are moistened. Fold in stiffly beaten egg whites. Bake on hot griddle.

Low-Calorie Desserts

NO-CRUST APPLE PIE
(123 calories per portion. Serves 7.)

2 egg yolks
1 1/2 teaspoons artificial sweetener
2 tablespoons cornstarch
1/4 teaspoon allspice
1/4 teaspoon cloves
1/4 teaspoon nutmeg
1/4 teaspoon cinnamon

Instructions: Put all ingredients into the bowl of an electric blender and blend 2 seconds. Add 7 large apples, peeled and cored. Blend until the apples are minced fine by beater blades. Grease a pie plate, and fill with the apple mixture. (No pie crust is required.) Bake in a 350° oven for 30 minutes. Cover the pie with the following meringue:

2 egg whites
4 tablespoons powdered dry skim milk
1/2 teaspoon lemon extract
1/2 teaspoon vanilla extract
1/2 teaspoon artificial sweetener

Instructions: Beat whites until stiff peaks form adding all the other ingredients halfway through the beating. Spread the stiff meringue on pie, and brown in a 350° oven for 10 minutes, until lightly brown.

CRUSTLESS PEACH DESSERT PIE
(112 calories per serving. Serves 6.)

6 dietetic peach halves
1 cup low calorie dessert whip
2 envelopes lemon or strawberry D-Zerta

Instructions: Place the peach halves, rounded side up, in a 9-inch pie plate. Whip the dessert topping until stiff, adding a few drops of non-caloric liquid sweetener if you prefer. Cover the peach halves with the whipped topping. Prepare the gelatin according to package directions and chill in refrigerator until it takes on the consistency of egg white. Spoon semi-congealed gelatin over the whipped topping and peaches to cover completely. Chill until firm. Cut between peach halves into wedges to serve as you would a pie.

NO-CRUST PUMPKIN PIE
(68 calories per serving. Makes 8 portions.)

1 1-pound can pumpkin
2 tablespoons liquid artificial sweetener
1/2 teaspoon salt
1/2 teaspoon cinnamon
1/2 teaspoon ground ginger
1/4 teaspoon allspice
1/4 teaspoon ground cloves
2 eggs, slightly beaten
1 3/4 cups skim milk or reconstituted dry skim milk
2 egg whites

Instructions: Mix pumpkin, liquid sweetener, and all the seasonings well. Stir into the beaten eggs. Add milk, gradually, mixing well each time. Beat egg whites until stiff peaks form. Fold into pumpkin mixture. Pour into a greased baking dish and bake in a 375° oven for approximately 45–50 minutes until center tests done.

PINEAPPLE CREME
(51 calories per serving. Makes 8 portions.)

1 package dietetic vanilla pudding
1 cup skim milk
1 tablespoon unflavored gelatin
2 eggs, separated
1 teaspoon artificial liquid sweetener
1/2 teaspoon pineapple extract
1 small can (10 oz.) dietetic crushed pineapple, drained
1/2 cup ice water
1/2 cup powdered skim milk, dry

Instructions: Cook the pudding according to package directions, using skim milk. Soften the unflavored gelatin in 2 tablespoons cold water. Just before the pudding comes to a boil, add the slightly beaten egg yolks, stirring vigorously. Now add the gelatin. Bring to a boil and remove from heat, stirring well. Cool. Now stir in the liquid sweetener, the extract, and the drained pineapple. Beat egg whites until stiff peaks form. Add the dry milk powder to the ice water and beat to the consistency of whipped cream. Fold both the beaten whites and the beaten whipped milk powder into the cooled pudding. Turn into a rinsed pudding mold or a bowl and chill until ready to serve.

OATMEAL DESSERT COOKIES
(54 calories per cookie. Makes 3 dozen cookies.)

1/2 cup vegetable margarine
1 egg
1 level tablespoon dry sugar substitute
1 1/2 cups cake flour
1/2 teaspoon baking soda
1/4 teaspoon salt
1 1/2 teaspoons cinnamon
1/2 teaspoon each of cloves, nutmeg, and allspice
1/2 cup liquid skim milk
2 teaspoons vanilla
2 cups quick rolled oats
1/4 cup unsweetened applesauce
1/4 cup chopped walnuts
1/2 cup raisins

Instructions: Cream the margarine until soft. Beat egg and sugar substitute together until a lemon color shows. Add to shortening and blend well. Sift together the cake flour, soda, salt, and spices. Add to the shortening mixture alternately with the skim milk. Add the vanilla. Blend in remaining ingredients. Preheat oven to 375°. Drop dough by teaspoons on an oiled cookie sheet. Bake 12 minutes until lightly brown.

BANANA BREAD OR CAKE
(49 calories per slice.)

4 medium ripe bananas, mashed
1 tablespoon granulated sugar substitute
2 eggs, well beaten
1 3/4 cups cake flour
3 teaspoons baking powder
1/4 teaspoon salt
1/4 teaspoon chopped nuts
1/2 teaspoon vanilla flavoring

Instructions: Sprinkle sugar substitute over bananas and stir until dissolved. Blend in beaten eggs. Sift the flour, baking powder, and salt together. Add the chopped nuts and vanilla. Blend thoroughly into banana mixture, but do not overbeat. Preheat oven to 350°. Pour batter into a greased loaf pan, which has been lightly dusted with flour. (A 4 x 7 inch pan works best.) Bake 25 minutes at 350°, then reduce heat to 300° and continue baking about 35 more minutes until center tests done. Cut each loaf into 20 slices.

FRESH STRAWBERRY-PINEAPPLE ROMANOFF
(74 calories per serving. Serves 8.)

2 cups fresh strawberries, washed and hulled
1 cup fresh pineapple, cubed
1 1/2 cups low calorie dessert topping, whipped
1/2 cup orange juice
1 ounce orange Curacao (or substitute orange extract)
1 teaspoon artificial liquid sweetener

Instructions: Combine orange juice, liquid sweetener, and Curacao or flavoring and pour over the berries and pineapple in a large bowl. Marinate at least 1 1/2 hours. Refrigerate until ready to serve. At serving time, place the bowl of fruit and a bowl of whipped low-calorie dessert topping on the table. Toss together at the table and spoon into dessert dishes for individual serving.

FRUIT WHIP
(51 calories per serving. Makes 6 portions.)

1 cup dietetic fruit salad, drained
1 large banana, peeled and cubed
1/2 cup ice water
1/2 cup dry skim milk powder
2 ounces raspberry dietetic gelatin
1/2 teaspoon artificial liquid sweetener
1/2 teaspoon lemon flavoring

Instructions: Arrange fruit in a glass bowl. Prepare the gelatin according to package directions. Add the liquid sweetener. Combine with the fruit and refrigerate until it begins to set. Beat the dry milk powder and the ice water together with an electric beater, adding an additional 1/2 teaspoon liquid sweetener and the lemon flavoring. Beat until peaks form, about 3 minutes. Stir into the fruit and gelatin mixture until thoroughly combined. Spoon into sherbet glasses and refrigerate until set.

Low-Calorie Snacks

SKIM MILK—MILK SHAKES

Place the following in a blender:
1/3 cup powdered skim milk
1/2 cup water, or a fruit juice
1/2 tray of the small ice cubes
5 to 8 frozen strawberries or equal blueberries, or any fruit (non sugared)
Artificial sugar to taste (such as Sugar Twin). You can make this thinner or thicker by adding or subtracting strawberries.
Portions: 1 milk, 2 fruit

WHEAT THIN HORS D'OEUVRE

Shavings of cheese in bowl surrounded by Wheat Thins.

FRENCH TOAST WITH STRAWBERRY TOPPING

Dip a slice of bread into a batter of :
1 egg, or egg substitute
2 tsp. water
1/8 tsp. monosodium-glutamate
1 tsp. sugar substitute
Brown on a non-stick skillet or use Pam or other non-stick.
Strawberry topping is prepared by mashing:
1/2 cup strawberries
1 tsp. sugar substitute
Few drops of vanilla

MIXED VEGETABLES

Steam cook frozen mixed vegetables. Wire steam baskets are generally available and fit in ordinary pans.
Sprinkle with powdered parmesan cheese.

RHUBARB

5 pounds raw rhubarb
1/4 cup water
1 capful lemon extract
7 tsp. sugar substitute

Instructions: Cut into 1 inch pieces. Boil rhubarb about 20 minutes in water slowly stirring occasionally. Add lemon extract and sugar substitute. Chill.

POPCORN

Pop corn using a minimum layer of vegetable oil, an ordinary thick aluminum pan works fine on high heat, add salt only.

VEGETABLE SOUP

Heat a small can of V-8 juice. The taste is potent and being hot encourages sipping.

BRUSSELS SPROUTS

Steam or pressure cook a bunch. Keep cool in refrigerator (Keeps several days). Nibble occasionally as is, or sprinkle parmesan cheese.

FRUIT SALAD

1 can unsweetened pineapple
2 apples
1/3 cup powdered milk
1/3 cup water
1 tbsp. sugar sweetener
2 tsp. lemon juice
1 tsp. vanilla

Instructions: Dice apples and combine with pineapple. Blend or whip remaining ingredients and pour apple-pineapple ring.

SHERBET

Pour can of any flavor non-caloric carbonated beverage into ice cube tray (small ice cubes). Place these ice cubes in blender with 1/3 cup non-fat dry milk and 1/3 cup of water.

OPTIMAL BUTTER SUBSTITUTE

(For use in diets where butter and other spreads cannot be used.)

Amount	Ingredient
1 tablespoon	cornstarch
2/3 cup	non-fat dry milk powder
1 teaspoon	salt
2 cups	corn oil
2/3 cup	water
	yellow food color
1 tablespoon	lemon juice

Instructions:

1. Sift cornstarch and instant dry milk powder and salt together in top of double boiler.

2. Combine lemon juice and water, gradually add to starch mixture, mixing until smooth.

3. Cook over boiling water, stirring constantly until mixture thickens, about 4 minutes. Remove from heat.

4. Add corn oil, 1/4 cup at a time, beating with rotary beater after each addition. Add coloring.

Do not use electric blender

1 tablespoon = 95 calories

This spreads well, but does not melt. Makes 1 pound 5 1/2 ounces per recipe.

Appendix C:
Food Cholesterol Levels

Avoid	Seek
Average American intake, 600–1500 mg/day cholesterol	300 mg/day
Saturated fats (animal origin)	Unsaturated fats (vegetable origin)
Creamy cheese, egg yolk, butter, pork, beef	Margarine*, grains, skim milk, up to 3 eggs per week, leafy vegetables, nuts, fish, poultry
Organ meats	Limit 4 oz. liver per week
Coconut, palm oil	Safflower, soybean, corn oil, whole grain cereals, fruit, non-fat milk, yogurt, graham crackers, roasted soybeans, nuts, raisins
Overeating	Roughage (whole grains, leafy vegetables)
Tension	Exercise

CHOLESTEROL LEVELS IN FOOD
(mg per 100 grams of food)

Food	mg	Food	mg
beef, raw	70	ice cream	45
brains, raw	2000	kidney, raw	375
butter	250	lamb, raw	70
caviar or roe	300	lard and other animal fats	95
cheese		liver, raw	300
Cheddar	100	lobster	200
cottage (creamed)	15	margarine	
cream	120	all vegetable fat	0
others (25–35%)	85	1/3 vegetable and	
		2/3 animal fat	65
cheese spreads	65	milk	
chicken, raw (no skin)	60	fluid, whole	11
crab	125	dried, whole	85
egg, whole	550	fluid, skim	3
white	0	mutton	65
egg, yolks		oysters	200
fresh	1500	pork	70
frozen	1280	shrimps	125
dried	2950	sweetbreads (thymus)	250
fish, steak or fillet	70	veal	90
heart, raw	150		

*Must have liquid corn, soy, or safflower oil as its principal ingredient.

LOW-FAT, LOW-CHOLESTEROL FOOD GUIDE

LOW-FAT
(less than 5 gm/serving)

Angel or sponge cake
bouillon, commercial beef or
  chicken broth and consomme
bread, commercial
buttermilk
carbonated beverages, fruit-
  flavored drinks
catsup, chili sauce
cereals
chicken, white meat, no skin (3 oz.)
cocoa powder
coffee, tea
cornstarch
cottage cheese, uncreamed
crackers, made without shortening,
  matzoh
egg white
fish (3 oz.)
bluefish, cod, haddock, pike,
  swordfish, clams, crab, oysters,

scallops, shrimp, tuna, fresh or
  water packed
flours
fruit and fruit juice (except
  avocados)
fruit ice
gelatin, flavored and unflavored
hard candy, marshmallows
herbs, spices
honey, molasses, syrups
jams, jellies, marmalades, preserves
macaroni, noodles, spaghetti
mustard, prepared
pickles
sherbet
skim milk
sugars
vegetables and vegetable juice
vinegars
yoghurt, made from skim milk

LOW-CHOLESTEROL
(less than 10 mg/serving)

angel cake
bouillon, clear broths
bread, commercial white and
  wholewheat
buttermilk
carbonated beverages, fruit-
  flavored drinks
catsup, chili sauce
cereals
cocoa powder
coffee, tea
cornstarch
cottage cheese, uncreamed
egg white
flours
fruit and fruit juices
fruit ice
gelatin, flavored and unflavored
hard candy, marshmallows
herbs, spices

honey, molasses, syrup
jams, jellies, marmalades, preserves
macaroni, noodles, spaghetti
margarine, all vegetable fat
mayonnaise (2 tablespoons)
mustard, prepared
oils, vegetable
peanut butter
pickles
potato chips
salad dressing, French or Italian
skim milk
sugars
vegetables and vegetable juices
vinegars

Appendix D:
Fitness
Testing Methods

Protocol for Astrand Test on
Bicycle Ergometer

Equipment needed:

1. Bicycle ergometer
2. Metronome
3. Stopwatch (2)
4. Stethoscope

Procedure:

1. Practice taking heart rate (HR).

2. Set the metronome for the appropriate cadence (100/min. for the Monarch ergometer to allow one beat for each pedal stroke at a pedalling rate of 50 cycles/min.)

3. Set the ergometer seat so that subject's leg is almost straight at the knee at the bottom of pedal stroke, with ball of feet on the pedal.

4. With the subject seated on the ergometer, but resting, take the H.R. for 30 seconds by the following procedure:

(a) With the stethoscope bell or diaphragm, search the area to left of the sternum for the most distinct heart sounds. Mark this area with a felt pen; (b) if no stethoscope is available, palpate the carotid pulse, just below the angle of the jaw (light pressure only). Start the watch as you count "zero" on the first beat.

5. Have the patient pedal without load until he can maintain the cadence precisely.

6. Set the work load estimated to produce a H.R. between 130–150 (for men, 900 Kg.M/min., and for women 600 Kg.M/min. are good starting points for average young men and women).

7. Begin timing when the load is set and subject begins the exercise bout. Keep it going for six minutes.

8. Take the H.R. for the last 30 seconds of each minute for the six minute workbout.

9. Use the mean H.R. recorded in the fifth and sixth minute as the working heart rate for that work load. If difference between the two rates exceeds 5 beats/min. prolong the workbout until a constant level is attained.

10. If H.R. is below 130, the load should be increased in successive six minute workbouts by 300 KgM/min. until H.R. rises between 130–150.

11. Plot H.R. and workload to determine Max VO_2 on chart.

12. If the subject is over 30 years of age, multiply the Max VO_2 by the correction factor, then multiply by 1000 to obtain the figure in milliliters.

13. To normalize for body size, maximal oxygen uptake (max VO_2) is divided by body weight in kilograms (1 kg. = 2.2 lbs.) and the final result of the test will be expressed as ml/02/kg min.

Table D-1:
Prediction of Maximal Oxygen Uptake from Heart Rate and Work Load on Bicycle Ergometer*

Applies to men. The value should be corrected for age, using the factor given in Table D-3.

Heart Rate	Maximal Oxygen Uptake Liters/min.					Heart Rate	Maximal Oxygen Uptake Liters/min.				
	300 kpm/min.	600 kpm/min.	900 kpm/min.	1200 kpm/min.	1500 kpm/min.		300 kpm/min.	600 kpm/min.	900 kpm/min.	1200 kpm/min.	1500 kpm/min.
120	2.2	3.5	4.8			148		2.4	3.2	4.3	5.4
121	2.2	3.4	4.7			149		2.3	3.2	4.3	5.4
122	2.2	3.4	4.6			150		2.3	3.2	4.2	5.3
123	2.1	3.4	4.6			151		2.3	3.1	4.2	5.2
124	2.1	3.3	4.5	6.0		152		2.3	3.1	4.1	5.2
125	2.0	3.2	4.4	5.9		153		2.2	3.0	4.1	5.1
126	2.0	3.2	4.4	5.8		154		2.2	3.0	4.0	5.1
127	2.0	3.1	4.3	5.7		155		2.2	3.0	4.0	5.0
128	2.0	3.1	4.2	5.6		156		2.2	2.9	4.0	5.0
129	1.9	3.0	4.2	5.6		157		2.1	2.9	3.9	4.9
130	1.9	3.0	4.1	5.5		158		2.1	2.9	3.9	4.9
131	1.9	2.9	4.0	5.4		159		2.1	2.8	3.8	4.8
132	1.8	2.9	4.0	5.3		160		2.1	2.8	3.8	4.8
133	1.8	2.8	3.9	5.3		161		2.0	2.8	3.7	4.7
134	1.8	2.8	3.9	5.2		162		2.0	2.8	3.7	4.6
135	1.7	2.8	3.8	5.1		163		2.0	2.8	3.7	4.6
136	1.7	2.7	3.8	5.0		164		2.0	2.7	3.6	4.5
137	1.7	2.7	3.7	5.0		165		2.0	2.7	3.6	4.5
138	1.6	2.7	3.7	4.9		166		1.9	2.7	3.6	4.5
139	1.6	2.6	3.6	4.8		167		1.9	2.6	3.5	4.4
140	1.6	2.6	3.6	4.8	6.0	168		1.9	2.6	3.5	4.4
141		2.6	3.5	4.7	5.9	169		1.9	2.6	3.5	4.3
142		2.5	3.5	4.6	5.8	170		1.8	2.6	3.4	4.3
143		2.5	3.4	4.6	5.7						
144		2.5	3.4	4.5	5.7						
145		2.4	3.4	4.5	5.6						
146		2.4	3.3	4.4	5.6						
147		2.4	3.3	4.4	5.5						

*This table and Table D-2 from Astrand, I., *Physiologica Scandinavica* 49 (supp 169 1960), as modified by Astrand, P.O., in *Work Test with the Bicycle Ergometer* (Varberg, Sweden: Monark, 1965).

Table D-2:
Prediction of Maximal Oxygen
Uptake from Heart Rate and Work Load on
Bicycle Ergometer

Applies to women. The value should be corrected for age, using the factor given in Table D–3.

Heart Rate	Maximal Oxygen Uptake Liters/min.					Heart Rate	Maximal Oxygen Uptake Liters/min.				
	300 kpm/min.	450 kpm/min.	600 kpm/min.	750 kpm/min.	900 kpm/min.		300 kpm/min.	450 kpm/min.	600 kpm/min.	750 kpm/min.	900 kpm/min.
120	2.6	3.4	4.1	4.8		148	1.6	2.1	2.6	3.1	3.6
121	2.5	3.3	4.0	4.8		149		2.1	2.6	3.0	3.5
122	2.5	3.2	3.9	4.7		150		2.0	2.5	3.0	3.5
123	2.4	3.1	3.9	4.6		151		2.0	2.5	3.0	3.4
124	2.4	3.1	3.8	4.5		152		2.0	2.5	2.9	3.4
125	2.3	3.0	3.7	4.4		153		2.0	2.4	2.9	3.3
126	2.3	3.0	3.6	4.3		154		2.0	2.4	2.8	3.3
127	2.2	2.9	3.5	4.2		155		1.9	2.4	2.8	3.2
128	2.2	2.8	3.5	4.2	4.8	156		1.9	2.3	2.8	3.2
129	2.2	2.8	3.4	4.1	4.8	157		1.9	2.3	2.7	3.2
130	2.1	2.7	3.4	4.0	4.7	158		1.8	2.3	2.7	3.1
131	2.1	2.7	3.4	4.0	4.6	159		1.8	2.2	2.7	3.1
132	2.0	2.7	3.3	3.9	4.5	160		1.8	2.2	2.6	3.0
133	2.0	2.6	3.2	3.8	4.4	161		1.8	2.2	2.6	3.0
134	2.0	2.6	3.2	3.8	4.4	162		1.8	2.2	2.6	3.0
135	2.0	2.6	3.1	3.7	4.3	163		1.7	2.2	2.6	2.9
136	1.9	2.5	3.1	3.6	4.2	164		1.7	2.1	2.5	2.9
137	1.9	2.5	3.0	3.6	4.2	165		1.7	2.1	2.5	2.9
138	1.8	2.4	3.0	3.5	4.1	166		1.7	2.1	2.5	2.8
139	1.8	2.4	2.9	3.5	4.0	167		1.6	2.1	2.4	2.8
140	1.8	2.4	2.8	3.4	4.0	168		1.6	2.0	2.4	2.8
141	1.8	2.3	2.8	3.4	3.9	169		1.6	2.0	2.4	2.8
142	1.7	2.3	2.8	3.3	3.9	170		1.6	2.0	2.4	2.7
143	1.7	2.2	2.7	3.3	3.8						
144	1.7	2.2	2.7	3.2	3.8						
145	1.6	2.2	2.7	3.2	3.7						
146	1.6	2.2	2.6	3.2	3.7						
147	1.6	2.1	2.6	3.1	3.6						

Table D-3:
Correction Factors for Predicted Maximal Oxygen Uptake

Age	Factor	Max. heart rate	Factor
15	1,10	210	1,12
25	1,00	200	1,00
35	0,87	190	0,93
40	0,83	180	0,83
45	0,78	170	0,75
50	0,75	160	0,69
55	0,71	150	0,64
60	0,68		
65	0,65		

The actual factor should be multiplied by the value that is obtained from Tables D–1 and D–2.

Norms for Maximum O2 Consumption (Aerobic Working Capacity)

WOMEN

Age	Low	Fair	Average	Good	High
20-29	1.69	1.70-1.99	2.00-2.49	2.50-2.79	2.80+
	28	29-34	35-43	44-48	49+
30-39	1.59	1.60-1.89	1.90-2.39	2.40-2.69	2.70+
	27	28-33	34-41	42-47	48+
40-49	1.49	1.50-1.79	1.80-2.29	2.30-2.59	2.60+
	25	26-31	32-40	41-45	46+
50-65	1.29	1.30-1.59	1.60-2.09	2.10-2.39	2.40+
	21	22-28	29-36	37-41	42+

MEN

Age	Low	Fair	Average	Good	High
20-29	2.79	2.80-3.09	3.10-3.69	3.70-3.99	4.00+
	38	39-43	44-51	52-56	57+
30-39	2.49	2.50-2.79	2.80-3.39	3.40-3.69	3.70+
	34	35-39	40-47	48-51	52+
40-49	2.19	2.20-2.49	2.50-3.09	3.10-3.39	3.40+
	30	31-35	36-43	44-47	48+
50-59	1.89	1.90-2.19	2.20-2.79	2.80-3.09	3.10+
	25	26-31	32-39	40-43	44+
60-69	1.59	1.60-1.89	1.90-2.49	2.50-2.79	2.80+
	21	22-26	27-35	36-39	40+

Flexibility Evaluation

The following is to aid the physician in determining the patient's flexibility.

(a) Anatomical position is the starting position. Range of motion is measured with the tailbone as zero degree and the cranium as 180 degrees. Rotating motions are from the mid-sagittal plane (bisecting body into equal right and left sides) as zero degrees and the lateral plane as 180 degrees.

(b) All ranges are expressed as passive range of motion.

(c) The scale is divided into units of 10 degrees. Range of motion is recorded by filling in the area of range directly on attached sketch with date and examiner's initials.

(d) Use of same sheet for subsequent tests is recorded and dated accordingly.

(e) Retrogression is marked by diagonal lines over area of previous test and dated.

(f) If position is other than sketched, indicate S for supine, and P for prone.

SHOULDER

Flexion	0–90
Fl. & Rotation of scapula	90–180
Ext. & Rotation of scapula	180–90
Extension	90–50

SHOULDER

Abduction	0–90
Abd. & Rot. scapula	90–180
Add. & Rot. scapula	180–90
Abduction	90–0

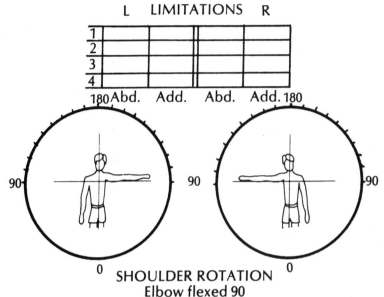

SHOULDER ROTATION
Elbow flexed 90

Ext. Rot.	0-90
Int. Rot.	0-90

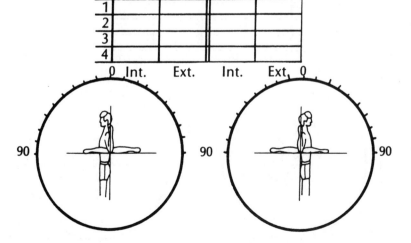

ELBOW

Flexion	0-145-160
Extension	160-145-0

L   **LIMITATIONS**   R

	Flex.	Ext.	Flex.	Ext.
1				
2				
3				
4				

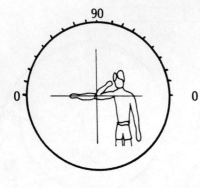 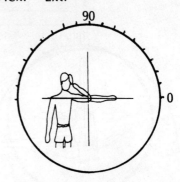

RADIO-ULNAR

Pronation	0-90
Supination	0-90

L   **LIMITATIONS**   R

	Sup.	Pron.	Sup.	Pron.
1				
2				
3				
4				

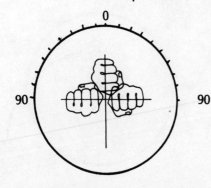 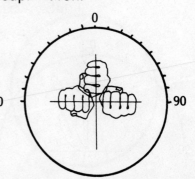

WRIST (flexion)

Dorsal Fl.	0-70
Volar Fl.	0-90

	L	LIMITATIONS		R	
1					
2					
3					
4					
	Dor.	Vol.		Dor.	Vol.

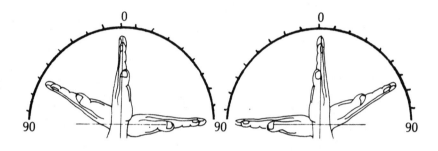

WRIST

Abduction	0-25
Abduction	0-55-65

	L	LIMITATIONS		R	
1					
2					
3					
4					
	Rad.	Uln.		Rad.	Uln.

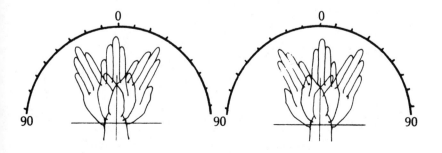

FINGERS MP

| Flexion | 0-90 |
| Extension | 0-20-30 |

L		L		R		R	
1 (II)		1 (III)		1 (II)		1 (III)	
2		2		2		2	
3		3		3		3	
4		4		4		4	
1		1(V)		1 (IV)		1 (V)	
2		2		2		2	
3		3		3		3	
4		4		4		4	
Fl.	Ext.	Fl.	Ext.	Fl.	Ext.	Fl.	Ext.

FINGERS I.P. PROX.

| Flexion | 0-120 |
| Extension | 120-0 |

LIMITATIONS

L				R			
1 (II)		(III)		(II)		(III)	
2							
3							
4							
1(IV)		(V)		(IV)		(V)	
2							
3							
4							
Fl.	Ext.	Fl.	Ext.	Fl.	Fl.	Ext.	Ext.

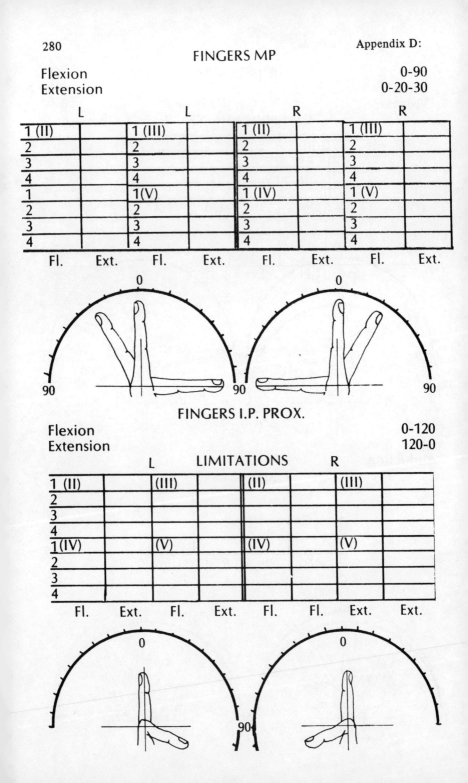

FINGERS I.P. DISTAL

Flexion	0-80
Extension	80-0

LIMITATIONS

	L				R			
1(II)		(III)		(II)		(III)	
2							
3							
4							
1(IV)		(V)		(IV)		(V)	
2							
3							
4							
	Fl.	Ext.	Fl.	Ext.	Fl.	Ext.	Fl.	Ext.

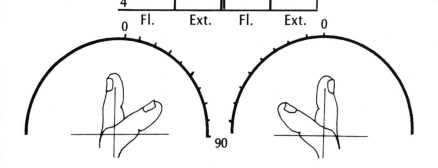

THUMB M.P.

Flexion	0-60-70
Extension	70-60-0

LIMITATIONS

	L		R	
1				
2				
3				
4				
	Fl.	Ext.	Fl.	Ext.

THUMB I.P.

Flexion   0-90
Extension   90-0

LIMITATIONS

	L			R	
1					
2					
3					
4					
	Fl.	Ext.	Fl.	Ext.	

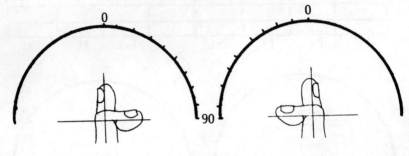

HIP

Fl. (str. knee)   0-90
Fl. (bent knee)   0-115-125
Extension   0-10-15
Ext. & Lumbar   0-15-45

SPINE
LIMITATIONS
Flexion (str. knee)

	L			R	
1					
2					
3					
4					
	Fl.	Ext.	Fl.	Ext.	

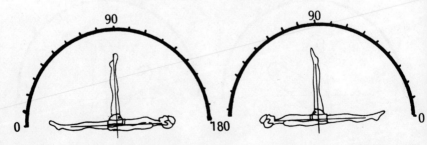

Flexion (Bent knee)

	L			R	
1					
2					
3					
4					
	Fl.	Ext.	Fl.	Ext.	

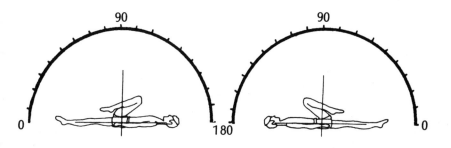

EXTENSION

	L			R	
1					
2					
3					
4					
	Ext.	F&L	Ext.	F&L	

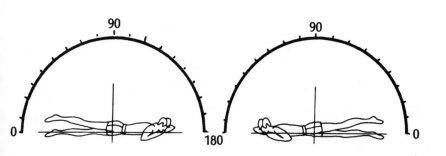

HIP

Abduction 0-45
Abduction 0-45

LIMITATIONS

	L		R	
1				
2				
3				
4				
	Abd.	Add.	Abd.	Add.

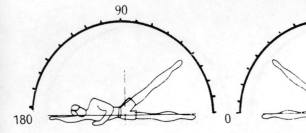
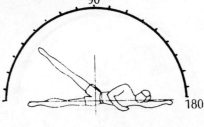

HIP (Bent Knee Prone)

Ext. Rot. 0-45
Int. Rot. 0-45

LIMITATIONS

	L		R	
1				
2				
3				
4				
	Int.	Ext.	Int.	Ext.

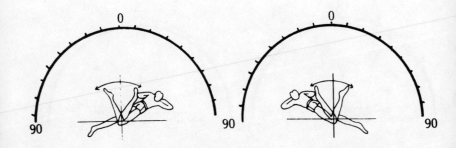

KNEE

| Flexion (prone) | 0-120-130 |
| Extension | 130-120-0 |

LIMITATIONS

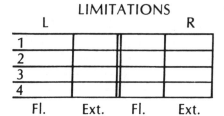

	L		R	
1				
2				
3				
4				
	Fl.	Ext.	Fl.	Ext.

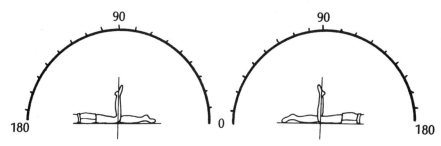

ANKLE

| Flexion | 0-20 |
| Extension | 0-45 |

LIMITATIONS

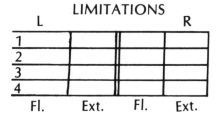

	L		R	
1				
2				
3				
4				
	Fl.	Ext.	Fl.	Ext.

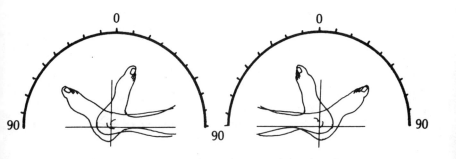

FOOT

Eversion	0-25
Inversion	0-35

LIMITATIONS

	L			R	
1					
2					
3					
4					
	Ev.	Inv.	Ev.	Inv.	

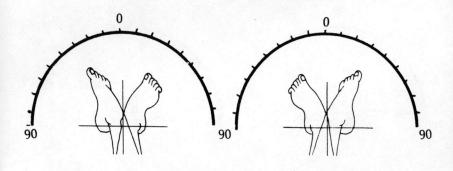

TOES M.P.

Flexion	0-25-35
Extension	0-80

LIMITATIONS

	L			R	
1					
2					
3					
4					
	Fl.	Ext.	Fl.	Ext.	

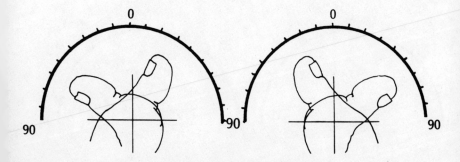

Source Notes

1. Walker, W. J. 1976. *Success story: The program against major cardiovascular risk factors. Geriat.* 31:97–104.
2. Lamb, L. E. 1975. *Your heart and how to live with it.* New York: New American Library.
3. Elrick, H., and Riffenburgh, R. 1974. Euexia (optimal health): body weight, in *San Diego Biomedical Symposium,* p. 41–6.
4. Stamler, J. 1967. *Lectures on preventative cardiology.* New York: Greene & Stratton.
5. White, L. S. 1975. How to improve the public's health. *N. Eng. J. Med.* 293 (15):773–74.
6. Johnson, W. R., and Buskirk, E. R. 1974. *Science and medicine of exercise and sport.* New York: Harper & Row.
7. Cooper, K. A. 1970. *The new aerobics.* New York: Bantam Books.
8. Hockey, R. V. 1973. *Physical fitness: The pathway to healthful living.* St. Louis: C. V. Mosby Company.
9. Morehouse, L. E. 1975. *Total fitness in 30 minutes a week.* New York: Simon & Schuster.
10. Skinner, J. S.; Holloszy, J. O.; and Cureton, T. K. 1964. Effects of a program of endurance exercises on physical work. *Am. J. Car.* 14:747.
11. Boyer, J. and Katsch, F. 1970. Exercise therapy in hypertensive men. *J.A.M.A.* 21: 10.
12. Hellerstein, H. K. A primary and secondary coronary prevention program in *Prevention of ischemic heart disease.* Raab, W., ed. Springfield: Charles C. Thomas.
13. Lamb, L. E. 1975. *Your heart and how to live with it.* New York: New American Library.
14. Miller, B., and Galton, L. 1972. *Freedom from heart attack.* New York: Simon & Schuster.
15. Naughton, J., and McCoy, J. F. 1966. Observations on the relationship of physical activities of the serum cholesterol concentration of healthy men and cardiac patients. *J. Chronic Dis.* 10: 727.
16. Mann, B. V., et al. 1969. Exercise to prevent coronary disease. *Am. J. Med.* 46: 12.
17. Golding, L. A. 1961. Effects of physical training upon total serum cholesterol levels. *Res. Quart.* 32: 499.
18. Cantoni, A. 1964. Physical effort and its effects on reducing alimentary hyperlipemia. *J. Sports Med. & Phys. Fit.* 4: 32.
19. Holloszy, J. O. 1975. Adaptation of skeletal muscle to endurance exercise. *Med. & Sci. in Sports.* 7(3): 155–64.
20. Kuntzelman, C. T., ed. 1971. *Physical fitness encyclopedia.* Emmaus, Pa.: Rodale Press, Inc.
21. Handler, P., ed. 1970. *Biology and the future of man.* London: Oxford University Press.
22. Selye, H. 1956. *The stress of life.* New York: McGraw-Hill Book Company.
23. Mann, C. 1959. Music and exercise as a form of psychotherapy.

Psychoan. Rev. 37: 143–55.

24. Ismail, Ah. H., and Trachtman, L. E. 1973. Jogging the imagination. *Psychology Today.*

25. Hammond, E. C. 1964. Some preliminary findings on physical complaints from a prospective study of 1,064,004 men and women. *A.J.P.H.* 54 (1):11–23.

26. Cooper, K. A. 1974. *Summary of tests on 15,000 clients.* Read at conference at the Aerobics Center, Dallas, Texas.

27. *Heart Facts.* 1976. New York: American Heart Association.

28. Dehn, M. M., and Bruce, R. A. 1962. Variations in maximal oxygen uptake with age and activity. *J. Appl. Physiol.* 33 (6).

29. Karvonen, J. J. 1956. Survival of Finnish champion skiers. *Duodicim.* 72: 893.

30. Fox, S. M.; Naughton, J. P.; and Haskell, W. L. 1971. Physical activity and the prevention of coronary heart disease. *Acta. Clin. Res.* 3:424–32; Morris, J. N.; Chave, S. P. W.; Adam, C.; Sirey, C.; and Epstein, L. 1973. Vigorous exercise in leisure time and the incidence of coronary heart disease. *Lancet.* 1:333–39; Sanne, H. 1973. Exercise tolerance and physical training of new selected patients after myocardial infarction. *Acta. Med. Scand. Supp., 551.*

31. Bruce, R. A. 1972. Multistage treadmill test of submaximal and maximal exercise. *Exercise testing and training of apparently healthy individuals.* New York: American Heart Association.

32. Brozek, J., and Keys, A. 1951. The evaluation of leanness-fatness in man: norms and interrelationships. *British Journal of Nutrition.* 5:194–206.

33. Sloan, A. W., Burt, J. J., and Blyth, C. S. 1962. Estimation of body fat in young women, *J. App. Phys.* 17:967070.

34. Astrand, P. O., and Rodahl, K. 1970. *Textbook of work physiology.* New York: McGraw-Hill Book Company.

35. Cooper, K. A. 1970. *New aerobics.* New York: Bantam Books.

36. Friedman, M., and Rosenaum, R. H. 1974. *Type A behavior and your heart.* New York: Alfred A. Knopf.

37. Astrand, P. O., and Rodahl, K. 1970. *Textbook of work physiology.* New York: McGraw-Hill Book Company, p. 362.

38. Cooper, K. A. 1970. *New aerobics.* New York: Bantam Books.

39. Bruce, R. A. 1972. *Exercise testing and training of apparently healthy individuals: A handbook for physicians.* New York: American Heart Association, p. 32.

40. Cureton, T. 1970. *Physical fitness workbook for adults.* Champaign, Ill.: Stipes Publishing Co., p. 116.

41. Cooper, K. A. 1968. *Aerobics.* New York: Bantam Books, p. 36.

42. Barnard, R. J. 1976. The heart needs warm-up time. *The physician and sportsmedicine,* p. 40.

43. See latest October issue of *Runner's World* for ratings of running shoes.

44. Zohman, L. R. 1974. *Beyond Diet . . . Exercise your way to fitness*

and heart health. New York: American Heart Association, p. 15.

45.   Bowerman, W. J. 1974. *Coaching track and field.* Boston: Houghton Mifflin Co., pp. 17–20.

46.   Jensen, C., and Fisher, G. 1972. *Scientific basis of athletic training.* Philadelphia: Lea & Febiger, p. 129.

47.   De Lorma, T. L., and Watkins, A. L. 1951. *Progressive resistance exercise.* New York: Appleton-Century Crofts.

48.   Kraux, Hans. 1956. *Principles and practice of therapeutic exercises.* Springfield, Mass.: Charles C. Thomas.

49.   Dayton, O. W. *Training and conditioning.* New York: The Ronald Press Co., p. 349.

50.   Williams, R. J. 1973. *Nutrition against disease.* New York: Bantam Books.

51.   Goodhart, R. S. 1973. Criteria of an adequate diet, in *Modern nutrition in health and disease.* Goodhart, R. S., and Shils, M. E., eds. Philadelphia: Lea & Febiger.

52.   Power, L. 1976. As physicians, we are too lax on nutrition. *Medical Opinion,* 5 (2): February.

53.   Miller, B. F., and Galton, L. 1972. *Freedom from heart attacks.* New York: Simon & Shuster; Yudkin, J. 1974. Dietary carbohydrate and serum cholesterol. *Lancet* 1:1007–18.

54.   Levy, R. I., and Ernest, H. Diet, Hyperlipoproteinemia and atherosclerosis, in *Modern nutrition, in health and disease.* Goodhart, R. S., and Shils, M. E., eds. Philadelphia: Lea & Febiger.

55.   Grande, F. 1974. Diet and atherosclerosis. *S.A. Med. J.* 48 (39): 1660–68.

56.   Elrick, H. 1974. Exercise and longevity, in *The Complete Runner.* Mountain View, Calif.: World Publications, pp. 168–71.

57.   Hardinge, M. G., and Crooks, H. 1963. Non-flesh dietaries: II. scientific literature. *J. Am. Diet. Ass'n.* 43: 550.

58.   Skrimshaw, N. S., et al. 1961. All vegetable protein mixtures for human feedings. *Am. J. Clin. Nutr.* 9:196.

59.   Kirkeby, K. 1966. Blood lipids, lipoproteins, and proteins in vegetarians. *Acta. Med. Scand.* 179: Suppl. 443.

60.   Mann, G. V. 1976. *The Physician and Sportsmedicine,* p. 87; Refsum, H. E. 1974. *J. Clin. & Lab.* 33:274–84; Nelson, R. A. 1975. What should athletes eat? *The Physician and Sportsmedicine,* pp. 66–72; Leaf, A. 1975. *Youth in old age.* New York: McGraw-Hill Book Company.

61.   Nelson, R. A. 1975. What should athletes eat? *The Physician and Sportsmedicine,* pp. 66–72.

62.   Caldwell, J. R. 1976. Perspectives in hypertensions. *Geriat.* vol. 31, p. 46–47.

63.   Kark, R. M., and Oyama, J. H. 1973. Nutrition and cardiovascular renal diseases, in *Modern nutrition and health disease.* Philadelphia: Lea & Febiger.

64.   Epstein, S. S. 1974. Environmental determinants of human cancer. *Cancer Res.* 34:2425–35.

291

65. Wynder, E. L. 1975. Introductory remarks in nutrition in the causation of cancer. *Cancer Res.* 35(11):3238; Wynder, E. L., and Reddy, B. S. 1974. Metabolic epidemiology of colo-rectal cancer. *Cancer Res.* 34 (suppl.):801–6; Wynder, E. L. 1975. The epidemiology of large bowel cancer, *Cancer Res.* 35:3388–94.
66. Doll, R. 1976. Epidemilogy of cancer: current perspectives. *Am. J. of Eped.* 104 (4): 396–404.
67. Shils, M. E. 1973. Nutrition and neiplasia, in *Modern nutrition in health and disease.* Philadelphia: Lea & Febiger.
68. Lowenfels, A. B., and Anderson, M. E. 1977. Diet and cancer. *Cancer.* 39 (4): 1809–14.
69. Phillips, R. L. 1975. Role of lifestyle and dietary habits in risk of cancer among Seventh-day Adventists. *Cancer Res.* 35:1513–220.
70. Wynder, E. L. 1976. Nutrition and cancer. *Federation proceedings* 35(6): 1309–15.
71. Addis, T. 1949. *Glomerular nephritis: diagnosis and treatment.* New York: MacMillan Co.
72. Giovanetti, S., and Maggiore, Q. 1964. A low-nitrogen diet with proteins of high biological value for severe chronic uremia. *Lancet.* 1:1000; Franklin, S., et al. 1967. Use of balanced low-protein diet in chronic renal failure. *AMA* 202:477; Maddock, R. K., et al. 1968. Low-protein diets in management of renal failure. *Ann. Int. Med.* 69:1003.
73. Shaw, A. F., et al. 1965. The treatment of chronic renal failure by a modified Giovanetti diet. *Quart. J. Med.* 34:237.
74. Goleman, Daniel. 1976. Meditation helps break the stress spiral. *Psychology Today.* 9 (9): 82–93.
75. Holmes, T. 1974. How change can make us ill. *Stress.* Blue Cross.
76. Lowen, Alexander. 1975. *Pleasure, a creative approach to life.* New York: Penguin Books, Inc.
77. Jacobsen, Edmund. 1934. *You must relax.* New York: McGraw-Hill Book Company.
78. Nell, Renee. 1971. Guidance through dreams, in *Ways of growth.* New York: Pocket Books.
79. Hammond, E. Cuyler. 1964. Some preliminary findings on physical complaints from a prospective study of 1,064,004 men and women. *Am. J. Pub. Health.* 54 (1): 11–23.
80. Benson, Herbert. 1974. Your innate asset for combatting stress. *Harv. Bus. Rev.* 52 (4): 49–60.
81. Goleman, D. 1976. Meditation helps break the stress spiral. *Psychology Today.* 9 (9): 82–93.
82. Naranjo, C. and Ornstein, R. E. 1972. *On the psychology of meditation.* New York: The Viking Press.
83. Latner, Joel. 1974. *The Gestalt therapy book.* New York: Bantam Books.
84. Robbins, J. and Fisher, D. 1973. *How to make and break habits.* New York: Peter H. Wyden, Inc.
85. *Act. Physiol. Scand.* 49 (Supp 169) 1960. p. 45–60.

About the Authors

Harold Elrick, M.D., FACP

Dr. Elrick received his M.D. degree at Harvard Medical School and had post-graduate training at the Massachusetts General Hospital, the Universities of Lund and Uppsala (Sweden), and McGill University. He was on the medical faculty of Harvard and Colorado Universities. He is currently in private practice specializing in preventive medicine, nutrition, and physical fitness and is the Director of the Foundation for Optimal Health and Longevity in San Diego, California. His interests include distance running, foreign languages, and sports.

James G. Crakes, Ph.D.

Dr. Crakes obtained his B.S., M.S., and Ph.D. degrees in Physical Education at the University of Oregon and a Physical Therapy certificate from New York University. He has held coaching and teaching positions at junior and senior high schools and for the past seventeen years has taught exercise physiology and coached track and field at the university level. Several of his athletes have won national championships and participated in the Olympic Games.

He is currently an Associate Professor at Point Loma College (San Diego).

Samuel J. Clarke, Jr., M.S.

Mr. Clarke obtained his B.S. in Psychology and M.S. in Exercise Physiology at the University of Washington. He has held training management positions with the Boeing Company and the Unigard Insurance Corporation. Now a training consultant, he gives programs in management and physical fitness for industries and community colleges in the Seattle area. His hobbies and interests are distance running, creating optimal recipes, and producing educational television programs.

Index

Other World Publications Books on Health and Fitness

FITNESS AFTER FORTY   *Hal Higdon*

DR. SHEEHAN'S MEDICAL ADVICE   *George Sheehan, M.D.*
For Runners and Other Athletes

BASIC FITNESS GUIDE   *Joe Owens*

THE COMPLETE DIET GUIDE   *Edited by Hal Higdon*
For Runners and Other Athletes

SKIN CARE   *Cameron L. Smith, M.D.*
For Men and Women Outdoors

WORLD
World Publications
1400 Stierlin Road
Mountain View, CA 94043